Breast Cancer and Medical Imaging

Online at: https://doi.org/10.1088/978-0-7503-5709-8

IOP Series in Medical and Biological Image Analysis

Series Editor: Robert Koprowski PhD DSc, University of Silesia, Katowice, Poland

Editor Bio: Robert Koprowski, PhD, is a lecturer in the Department of Biomedical Computer Systems in Computer Science Institute at The University of Silesia, Katowice, Poland. His research interests include computer analysis and signal and biomedical image processing, as well as computer science technology in medicine and biotechnology. He is an author and co-author of 8 published books and has published over 140 papers.

Aims and Scope: The scope of this series involves the use of image analysis and processing methods in medicine and biology. New areas of medicine and biology in which image analysis and processing methods have not been used so far will be equally interesting to explore in this series - especially those operating automatically and repetitively in large patient populations. Additionally, any imaging method can be applied, starting with MRI through X-ray and ending with THV or other imaging methods that have not yet been invented. This series also includes works which are a combination of an engineer (algorithms for image analysis and processing) and a doctor (who verifies the practical clinical utility of the proposed image analysis and processing methods).

A full list of titles published in this series can be found here: https://iopscience.iop.org/bookListInfo/iop-series-in-medical-and-biological-image-analysis#series.

Breast Cancer and Medical Imaging

Mohammed Erkhawan Hameed Rasheed
Mansour Youseffi
Biomedical and Electronics Engineering Department, Faculty of Engineering and Informatics, University of Bradford, Bradford, United Kingdom

IOP Publishing, Bristol, UK

ISBN   978-0-7503-5709-8 (ebook)
ISBN   978-0-7503-5707-4 (print)
ISBN   978-0-7503-5710-4 (myPrint)
ISBN   978-0-7503-5708-1 (mobi)

DOI   10.1088/978-0-7503-5709-8

Version: 20240301

IOP ebooks

British Library Cataloguing-in-Publication Data: A catalogue record for this book is available from the British Library.

Published by IOP Publishing, wholly owned by The Institute of Physics, London

IOP Publishing, No.2 The Distillery, Glassfields, Avon Street, Bristol, BS2 0GR, UK

US Office: IOP Publishing, Inc., 190 North Independence Mall West, Suite 601, Philadelphia, PA 19106, USA

To my late parents, Hameed Rasheed, and Sophia Kareem, who taught me to read and write when I was a child before starting school and instilled in me values and the first lessons of knowledge and wisdom. 'And say: My Lord, have mercy upon them as they raised me up when I was little'.

—M E H Rasheed

Contents

Preface

This book starts with a systematic coverage of the review literature on the topic of breast cancer including the various stages of the disease, the risk factors, as well as breast cancer prevention strategies and control. This work also discusses the various types of breast cancer and the symptoms of the disease followed by the available treatments including surgery, chemotherapy, radiotherapy, in addition to hormone treatment and targeted therapy. The work similarly presents the various complementary and alternative natural remedies used around the world to treat the disease and help patients with the symptoms including palliative care. This book presents a detailed explanation of the topics of breast cancer and almost all the medical imaging modalities that are used for breast cancer screening, diagnosis and treatment monitoring, in simple, easy to understand language with detailed clinical case studies supported by detailed medical images and analysis. The medical imaging modalities discussed in this work include non-ionising imaging modalities such as ultrasound and magnetic resonance imaging (MRI), as well as imaging with ionising radiation such as conventional X-ray imaging, mammography, computed tomography (CT) imaging, and nuclear medicine imaging including positron emission tomography (PET) scans and single-photon emission computerised tomography (SPECT) scans, in addition to hybrid imaging modalities such as PET/CT and PET/MR. This book then covers various case studies carried out using appropriate medical imaging techniques with clear images and image analysis related to various cancerous tissues with discussions on the topics of clinical genetics and genetic counselling related to this work, as well as the use of artificial intelligence (AI) for the enhancement of breast cancer imaging. These are discussed sufficiently in detail and depth with good understanding and in relation to the topics discussed in this work, and concluded appropriately with many useful and up to date references. This book is written in good scientific and technical English and some parts of the work, such as the results of the clinical cancer case studies, have already been presented at scientific conferences and published in the form of journal articles in Scopus indexed peer-reviewed journals, such as the Institute of Electrical and Electronics Engineers (IEEE) Xplore and the American Institute of Physics (AIP) Conference Proceedings, as explained in each relevant chapter. In summary, this book represents the research conducted over many years in the areas of breast cancer, medical imaging and cancer genetics, and provides a detailed review of the topics of breast cancer and the current knowledge, practices and techniques used for various medical imaging modalities. Readers not familiar with such topics can use this book as a reference point to read, learn and practice, which will require detailed content and analysis as covered in each chapter. Providing detailed information is one of the important components of this book with the hope that it will be helpful for academics and researchers in the field, in addition to non-academics and for the benefit of the public.

Author biographies

Mohammed Erkhawan Hameed Rasheed, PhD

Dr Rasheed is a Chartered Scientist (CSci) and appointed Honorary Visiting Researcher within the Medical and Healthcare Technology Team in the Biomedical and Electronics Engineering Department, Faculty of Engineering and Informatics, University of Bradford, Bradford, UK. He works as the Principal Investigator (PI) in Clinical Cancer Research on clinical case studies of various cancer types with focus on genetic testing, medical imaging and treatments. He is also the Research Scientist in charge of investigating artificial intelligence (AI) and machine learning techniques for the enhancement of medical imaging modalities used for breast cancer and other types of cancer. He holds a PhD in Medical and Healthcare Technology from the University of Bradford, and he is a Fellow of the Institute of Biomedical Science.

Mansour Youseffi, PhD

Dr Youseffi is a Reader in Biomaterials and Admission Tutor for the undergraduate and postgraduate MSc programmes within the Biomedical and Electronics Engineering Department, Faculty of Engineering and Informatics, University of Bradford, Bradford, UK. He lectures in the following modules as the module leader: Materials Science and Engineering, Rehabilitation and Prosthetics, Functional Anatomy and Human Physiological Measurements, Biomaterials with Implant Design and Technology, Clinical Biomechanics, Cell and Tissue Biology, Regenerative Medicine, and Design Build and Test. He holds a PhD in Engineering from Loughborough University of Technology, Loughborough, UK and he is a Registered Practitioner and Fellow of the Higher Education Academy.

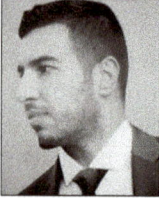

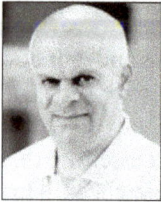

List of abbreviations

AIs	aromatase inhibitors
AI	artificial intelligence
ALND	axillary lymph node dissection
ATM	ataxia telangiectasia mutated
BARD1	brca1 associated ring domain 1
BCS	breast-conserving surgery
BI-RADS	breast imaging reporting and database systems
BRCA1	breast cancer gene 1
BRCA2	breast cancer gene 2
BRIP1	brca1 interacting protein c-terminal helicase 1
BSE	breast self-examination
BSP	breast screening programme
C+	contrast-enhanced
CAD	computer-aided detection
CAT	computerised axial tomography
CBE	clinical breast examination
CBs	cannabinoids
CC	craniocaudal
CDH1	cadherin-1
CHEK2	checkpoint kinase 2
CIS	carcinoma *in situ*
CXR	chest X-ray
DBT	digital breast tomosynthesis
DCIS	ductal carcinoma *in situ*
DD	dose-dense
DIBH	deep inspiration breath hold
DNA	deoxyribonucleic acid
ER+	oestrogen receptor-positive
FatSat	fat-saturated
FDA	food and Drug Administration
FDG	fluorodeoxyglucose
FFDM	full-field digital mammography
FSE	fast spin echo
G3	grade 3
HER2	human epidermal growth factor receptor 2
HRT	hormone replacement therapy
IBC	inflammatory breast cancer
ICB	immune checkpoint blockade
IDC	invasive ductal carcinoma
ILC	invasive lobular carcinoma
LCIS	lobular carcinoma *in situ*
MBI	molecular breast imaging
MDT	multidisciplinary team
MLO	mediolateral oblique
MpBC	metaplastic breast cancer
MRE11A	meiotic recombination 11 homolog a
NAC	neoadjuvant chemotherapy

NBN	nibrin
PA	posteroanterior
PALB2	partner and localiser of brca2
pH	power of hydrogen
PMS2	mismatch repair endonuclease
PTEN	phosphatase and tensin homolog
QOL	quality of life
RT	radiation therapy
SERMs	selective oestrogen receptor modulators
SFOV	scan field of view
SLNB	sentinel lymph node biopsy
STK11	serine/threonine kinase 11
T1W	t1-weighted
TNBC	triple-negative breast cancer
TNM	tumour node metastasis
TP53	tumour protein 53
TSE	turbo spin echo
ZW	zamzam water

Chapter 1

Introduction

According to the National Health Service (NHS), breast cancer is the most common type of cancer in the UK affecting mainly women aged 50 and above; however, it may also affect younger women [1]. Breast cancer is related to the uncontrolled growth of the breast cells and usually the disease is identified by a red appearance and swelling of the breast. However, many breast cancer patients do not have any noticeable symptoms in the early stages of the disease.

The common causes of breast cancer are due to gene mutations responsible for the normal healthy growth of the breast cells. For the breasts to function healthily, the old and damaged cells are continuously replaced by healthy cells. However, any changes in this process due to gene mutations may eventually lead to the out-of-control growth of the breast cells, which may lead to the formation of tumours. Gene mutations can be inherited (hereditary) or acquired (non-hereditary). Inherited gene mutations can be passed on from generation to generation, and a gene mutation that is linked to cancer may cause cancer to run in families. Only 5–10% of all cancers are thought to be hereditary [2, 3]. Women from families with a history of breast cancer are at a higher risk of developing the disease. The common hereditary breast cancers are linked to mutations in breast cancer gene 1 (BRCA1) and breast cancer gene 2 (BRCA2) [4]. BRCA1 and BRCA2 genes' function is to repair any breast cell damage and to maintain normal growth of the breasts. These mutated genes can be passed from parents (including relatives from both sides) to children. Whereas acquired gene mutations occur sometime during the lifetime of a person and can be caused by environmental factors or certain lifestyles. About 90–95% of all cancer cases are caused by acquired gene mutations and they tend to occur later in life compared to similar inherited cancer types [2, 3]. However, non-inherited genetic cancers may also appear to run in families when they have a shared environment or lifestyle behaviours [5, 6]. The stages of breast cancer are denoted by the number 0 and the Roman numerals I, II, III and IV. Stage 0 describes non-invasive breast cancer, which means cancer has not completely developed or

doi:10.1088/978-0-7503-5709-8ch1

spread into the surrounding areas of the breast, while stage IV is invasive, i.e., cancer has extended to other parts of the body [7].

Medical imaging tests such as mammography, in combination with clinical breast examination (CBE) and breast self-examination (BSE), contribute to the early detection of breast cancer before any symptoms appear in women who look healthy and are not suspected of having breast cancer. However, if any areas of concern during mammography are detected, breast ultrasound imaging (USI), breast magnetic resonance imaging (MRI), in addition to newer breast imaging tests such as molecular breast imaging (MBI) are recommended. A biopsy, i.e., a sample of breast cells that is taken from the patient and evaluated, is usually performed if a breast abnormality shows up, to determine whether or not breast cancer is present and also to find out if the disease has spread outside the breast (metastasis). Accurate breast cancer diagnosis, and staging (i.e., the degree of tumour spread) are used to guide treatment options and decisions for which several different imaging modalities are commonly used such as chest X-rays (CXR), computed tomography (CT) scans, bone scans, positron emission tomography (PET) scans or MRI scans. A PET scan is often combined with a CT scan, which is known as a PET/CT scan, to produce more detailed images and provide more accurate diagnoses [8].

There are various treatment choices available for breast cancer, and all depend on the type and stage of each case. A list of the main breast cancer treatments available include radiotherapy (RT), surgery, hormone replacement therapy (HRT), chemotherapy and biological therapy (targeted therapy). Radiotherapy and surgical treatments are local treatments, i.e., the breast tumour is treated with no damage to other parts of the body. On the other hand, HRT, chemotherapy and targeted therapy are systematic therapies, i.e., the drugs that are used to treat breast cancer can reach all parts of the body. Breast cancer patients often have one or a combination of these treatments depending on diagnosis and staging. The more the cancer has spread, the more treatment will likely be needed. A multidisciplinary team (MDT), which is a team of healthcare professionals and specialists who work together, is usually appointed to provide the best patient care and treatment [9]. Mammography, ultrasound, PET scan, CT scan, as well as breast MRI, play a vital role in breast cancer treatment response monitoring. Furthermore, monitoring tests are also used to check for any signs of recurrence in women who have had treatment for breast cancer. This work has focused on the following medical imaging modalities: X-ray, CT scan, mammography, ultrasound imaging, MRI, radionuclide imaging, PET scan, PET scan combined with CT scan, PET scan combined with MRI, single-photon emission computed tomography (SPECT) and SPECT scan combined with CT scan.

References

[1] NHS UK 2019 *Breast cancer in women* (NHS UK) (https://nhs.uk/conditions/breast-cancer/)
[2] Anand P, Kunnumakara A, Sundaram C, Harikumar K, Tharakan S, Lai O, Sung B and Aggarwal B 2008 Cancer is a preventable disease that requires major lifestyle changes *Pharm. Res.* **25** 2097–116

[3] Rizzolo P, Silvestri V, Falchetti M and Ottini L 2011 Inherited and acquired alterations in development of breast cancer *Appl. Clin. Genet.* **4** 145–58

[4] breastcancer.org 2018 *Genetics* (breastcancer.org) (https://breastcancer.org/risk/factors/genetics)

[5] National Cancer Institute 2017 *The genetics of cancer* (National Cancer Institute) (https://cancer.gov/about-cancer/causes-prevention/genetics)

[6] American Cancer Society 2020 *Family cancer syndromes* (American Cancer Society) (https://cancer.org/cancer/cancer-causes/genetics/family-cancer-syndromes.html)

[7] breastcancer.org 2018 *Breast cancer stages* (breastcancer.org) (https://breastcancer.org/symptoms/diagnosis/staging)

[8] NHS UK 2018 *PET scan* (NHS UK) (https://nhs.uk/conditions/pet-scan/)

[9] NHS UK 2016 *Treatment* (NHS UK) (https://nhs.uk/conditions/breast-cancer/treatment/)

Chapter 2

Breast cancer stages and risk factors

Similar to other types of cancer, breast cancer has become one of the major public health problems worldwide. Breast cancer is one of the four major cancer types in addition to lung cancer, prostate cancer and colorectal cancer, which drive global trends in the overall incidences of cancer cases [1]. For a better understanding of the elements associated with breast cancer, chapter 2 presents a review, discussing the anatomy of the breast, the stages of breast cancer, in addition to the risk factors of the disease.

2.1 Background

To gaining the right understanding of breast cancer, it is necessary to understand the aetiology of the breast and its formation. It is essential to understand the anatomy of the different parts of the human female breast in addition to its functions. Women's breasts are mostly made up of adipose tissue and glandular tissue. Adipose tissue is simply fat, while glandular tissue is the milk-producing tissue. Moreover, milk ducts transmit milk made in the glandular tissue to the nipple [2]. Clinical evidence has suggested that breast cancer can affect any part of the breast, including the ducts and tissue [3]. Breast cancer is described as a cancer type in which the breast cells start growing out of control and result in formation of a tumour. The severity of the disease is based on its various stages, mainly numbered from stages 0–IV. Stage IV is the most critical stage in which the tumour has turned malignant due to the growth of the cancer cells in the nearby tissues and it has spread to other parts of the body [4]. It can be identified that due to the emergence of novel screening technologies such as mammography, clinicians are able to detect the asymptomatic disease and symptoms associated with it rapidly and early, to provide timely intervention to affected women. Breast cancer is one of the most life-threatening types of cancers associated with the abnormal development of lumps in the breast. Identification of breast cancer is associated with a red and swollen appearance of the breast due to the uncontrolled growth of breast cells, which is referred to as malignance.

2-1

Investigations have further highlighted that when left unchecked for an assessment, these malignant cells can turn into conditions beyond the original tumour, spreading out to other body parts in a process called metastasis [5]. Breast cancer occurs due to changes in mutations of genes responsible for the regulation of growth of breast cells [6]. Such changes affect the functioning of the genes associated with retaining the health of the cells of the breast. The healthy functioning of the breast is associated with the orderly process of cell growth within the breast, i.e., automatic and continuous replacement of old cells by healthy ones. In cases where there is a change in such orderly processes and mutations start turning some of the genes on and off in a cell, this can lead to an uncontrollable division of breast cells. The increased production or overgrowth of cells in the breast eventually leads to the formation of tumours, which can be further categorised into benign or malignant [5].

2.2 Breast cancer stages

The stages of breast cancer are usually numbered 0, I, II, III and IV. Breast cancer staging depends on the severity of the cancer, i.e., the tumour size and whether the disease has hormone receptors as well as to what extent the cancer has spread to healthy tissues inside the breasts, the nearby lymph nodes, and the other body parts and organs. Stage IA and stage IB are the subdivisions of stage I. Stage IIA and stage IIB are the subdivisions of stage II. Furthermore, stage IIIA, stage IIIB and stage IIIC are the subdivisions of stage III [7]. The details of all these stages are given below.

2.2.1 Stage 0

Stage 0 is non-invasive breast cancer. In stage 0, cancer cells remain inside the affected area of the breast in the ducts of the breast tissue, without invasion to adjacent breast tissues. Stage 0 cancers are known as carcinoma *in situ*, i.e., cancer remains in the original place.

2.2.2 Stage I

Stage I is invasive breast cancer. However, it is an early stage breast cancer and cancer is contained to only the area where it first started in the breast tissue. Cancer may also be found in the lymph nodes near the breast. Stage I is subdivided into stage IA and stage IB.

2.2.2.1 Stage IA
Stage IA is invasive breast cancer. The tumour size is up to 2 cm in stage IA. Cancer has invaded the adjacent breast tissues but not outside the breast. In stage IA no cancer cells are found in the lymph nodes.

2.2.2.2 Stage IB
Stage IB is invasive breast cancer. In stage IB cancer cells of 0.2–2 mm in size are found in the axillary lymph nodes or the lymph nodes near the breastbone. A tumour of up to 2 cm in size may also be found in the breast.

2.2.3 Stage II

Stage II is invasive breast cancer. In stage II the cancer is bigger in size compared to stage I and it is found in a limited area of breast tissue. Cancer may also be found in the lymph nodes close to the breast. Stage II is subdivided into stage IIA and stage IIB.

2.2.3.1 Stage IIA

Stage IIA is invasive breast cancer. In stage IIA either no tumours are found in the breast, but cancer is found in the axillary lymph nodes, a tumour of up to 2 cm in size is found in the breast plus cancer is found in the axillary lymph nodes, or a tumour 2–5 cm in size is found in the breast but no cancer is found in the axillary lymph nodes.

2.2.3.2 Stage IIB

Stage IIB is invasive breast cancer. In stage IIB either a tumour of 2–5 cm in size is found in the breast in addition to groups of cancer cells of 0.2–2 mm in size found in the lymph nodes, a tumour of 2–5 cm in size is found in the breast and cancer has spread to the axillary lymph nodes or the lymph nodes near the breastbone, or a tumour bigger than 5 cm in size is found in the breast but no cancer is found in the axillary lymph nodes.

2.2.4 Stage III

Stage III is invasive breast cancer. In stage III the cancer is larger in size compared to stage I and stage II, and it has spread further into the breast tissue. Cancer is also found in the lymph nodes. Stage III is subdivided into stage IIIA, stage IIIB and stage IIIC.

2.2.4.1 Stage IIIA

Stage IIIA is invasive breast cancer. In stage IIIA, either no tumours are found, or a tumour of any size is found in the breast and cancer has spread to the axillary lymph nodes or the lymph nodes near the breastbone, a tumour of bigger than 5 cm in size is found in the breast and groups of cancer cells of 0.2–2 mm in size are found in the lymph nodes, or a tumour that is bigger than 5 cm in size is found in the breast and cancer has spread to the axillary lymph nodes or the lymph nodes close to the breastbone.

2.2.4.2 Stage IIIB

Stage IIIB is invasive breast cancer. In stage IIIB, a tumour of any size is found in the breast and cancer has reached the skin of the breast and the chest wall leading to ulcers and swelling. Cancer is also found in the axillary lymph nodes or the lymph nodes near the breastbone.

2.2.4.3 Stage IIIC

Stage IIIC is invasive breast cancer. Either no tumours or a tumour of any size is found in the breast and cancer has reached the skin of the breast and the chest wall leading to ulcers and swelling. Cancer is also found in the axillary lymph nodes, or the lymph nodes below or above the collar bone, or the lymph nodes close to the breastbone.

2.2.5 Stage IV

Stage IV is invasive breast cancer. Breast cancer is described as advanced or metastatic, i.e., cancer has spread from its origin to other body parts and organs such as the lungs and the bones in a process called metastasis. Bone metastasis is typically very common in breast cancer patients [7].

2.3 Breast cancer risk factors

Breast cancer has been identified as one of the most prevalent cancers in women worldwide including both the developed as well as the developing countries. However, and according to the World Health Organization (WHO) statistics, breast cancer is mostly referred to as a disease of the developed world, where people get the illness mainly due to environmental factors and lifestyle behaviours. In the United States of America, for example, highly prevalent rates of breast cancer are seen among white and black women, i.e., Europeans and Africans compared to the indigenous people of the continent such as the American Indian and Alaska Native women who have the lowest incidence rate [8]. In addition to race and ethnicity, other risk factors that are linked to breast cancer include obesity, high rates of smoking, high levels of alcohol consumption, reproductive history, and the increased use of hormone replacement therapy among American women. In comparison, breast cancer incidence rates in Asia are quite low with a breast cancer age-standardized incidence rate (ASR) in Asia of 29.1/100 000 compared to the US 92.9/100 000 [9]. Many factors such as the environment, eating habits, early marriage and pregnancy as well as early childbirth and prolonged breastfeeding among women in Asian countries are examined as key factors behind the comparatively lower prevalence rate. Other factors such as the trends of less smoking, less drinking of alcohol, less use of hormones and exercise have been recognised as key elements in Asian countries. Other risk factors that are linked to breast cancer include inheriting certain mutated genes. About up to 10% of breast cancer cases are believed to be directly caused by gene mutations that are hereditary and passed down from generation to generation. The most inherited breast cancers are linked to mutations in the genes, BRCA1 (BReast CAncer gene one) and BRCA2 (BReast CAncer gene two) [10]. Therefore, many factors affect breast cancer occurrence. Some of the factors can be changed, while some of the other factors cannot. For example, factors like obesity, lack of physical activity and drinking alcohol are among the factors that can be modified by choosing a healthy lifestyle. Other factors that cannot be modified include being a woman, age and genetics. The risk of developing breast cancer for females is 100 times larger than for males [11]. Reproductive factors, such as an early first menstrual cycle, late menopause and late age at first childbirth are highlighted as significant causes of breast cancer. Additionally, women taking hormone replacement therapy (HRT) and oral contraceptives are also at higher risk.

2.3.1 Age

The biggest breast cancer risk factor, after being a woman, is the aging process. Around 2 in 3 cases of invasive breast cancer are found amongst patients aged 50 years and older. However, around 1 in 8 cases of invasive breast cancer are found in patients under the age of 45 years. The reason behind this is that with the aging process the human body becomes weaker in repairing genetic damage and consequently there are higher chances for mutations to occur in the body [12, 13].

2.3.2 Family history and genetics

Genetic transmission is recognised as one of the most significant risk factors of breast cancer, and there is a higher risk of developing breast cancer in women who have close relatives diagnosed with the disease. About 5–10% cases of breast cancer are believed to be from abnormal genes passing from parents to children. Such genetic transfers can occur from close blood relatives, including relatives from both the father's side and the mother's side and, in general, about 15% of breast cancer patients have a family member diagnosed with the disease [11].

The common inherited cases of breast cancer are linked to mutations in BRCA1 and BRCA2 genes. Females with a BRCA1 mutation have about a 50–70% risk of developing breast cancer, while those with a BRCA2 mutation have about a 40–60% risk of developing the disease by age 70 [14]. BRCA1 and BRCA2 genes produce tumour suppressor proteins which help with repairing damaged DNA and keeping the breasts growing normally. Mutations in other genes, such as the PALB2 (Partner And Localiser of BRCA2) gene, are also associated with inherited breast cancers. PALB2 interacts with BRCA1 and BRCA2 at the DNA damage site to take part in repairing damaged DNA by homologous recombination (HR). PALB2 mutation is recognised for having a high risk of developing breast cancer, estimated at about 35% by age 70 [15].

Other high-risk gene mutations include the PTEN (phosphatase and tensin homologue deleted on chromosome 10) gene and TP53 (tumour protein 53) gene. The PTEN gene gives instructions for making a tumour suppressor enzyme that is found in almost all body tissues to regulate the normal growth of cells. On the other hand, the TP53 gene gives instructions for making a tumour suppressor protein called tumour protein p53, which also regulates the normal growth of cells. Women with a PTEN mutation have a lifetime risk of breast cancer of about 25–50%, while those with a TP53 mutation have the risk of getting any type of cancer of up to almost 100% [14].

Moderate to high risk gene mutations that are also associated with inherited breast cancers include the genes that help to repair damaged DNA, such as the ataxia-telangiectasia mutated (ATM) gene and the cadherin 1 (CDH1) gene [14]. Mutations to other genes such as the checkpoint kinase 2 (CHEK2) gene are considered moderate risk breast cancer genes [16]. CHEK2 is a tumour suppressor gene and it is also involved in repairing damaged DNA. In general, genetic testing is available to determine if a woman has BRCA1, BRCA2 or other gene mutations. In the UK, a referral is usually needed from a GP to a consultant specialist, so the patient can be seen and treated urgently [17].

2.3.3 Taking oral contraceptives

Taking oral contraceptives (birth control pills) is highly dominant among women worldwide to prevent pregnancy. Roughly 140 million women globally use some type of contraceptive pills, with 16 million being in the United States alone [18]. The various formulation types of such medicines also mediate the effects of such oral contraceptives on breast cancer. Clinical investigations have revealed that the use of oral contraceptives such as oestrogen at high dose, ethynodiol diacetate, in addition to other oral contraceptives, has been linked to a higher risk of breast cancer. However, low-dose oestrogen oral contraceptives are not subjected to a high risk of breast cancer [19]. Findings have also suggested that the risk of breast cancer associated with the use of hormonal contraceptives is further dependent on the duration of use. Therefore, the longer women take oral contraceptives, the higher their breast cancer risk. There is a 9% breast cancer risk for women taking contraceptives for less than a year and 38% for women taking contraceptives for 10 years and above [18].

2.3.4 Taking hormone replacement therapy (HRT)

Women take hormone replacement therapy (HRT) to help them in relieving the common symptoms of the menopause, such as vaginal dryness, mood swings, hot flushes, night sweats and reduced sex drive [20]. Using HRT formulations is also identified as a possible reason for women to be at a higher risk of developing breast cancer [21]. Breast cancer risks are typically greater among women using oestrogen–progestin formulations, than those using oestrogen-only formulations. High risks of breast cancer are further highlighted to be linked to HRT for oestrogen receptor positive breast cancers compared to oestrogen receptor negative breast cancers. Women going through hormone replacement therapy are subjected to an increased risk of breast cancer typically within two years of cessation. However, the relation-ship between HRT and the risks associated with breast cancer are also moderated by other factors such as menopause (mainly using HRT straight away after the onset of menopause) [22] in addition to a lean body mass; high mammographic breast densities are also linked to a higher breast cancer risk amongst women taking HRT [21].

2.3.5 Pregnancy history

Past studies have highlighted that full-term pregnancies before the age of 30 years decrease the long-term breast cancer risk amongst women. If women did not give birth in early life to their first child, then they are at a higher risk of getting breast cancer, compared to women who had their first child before the age of 30 years [23].

Pregnancy offers a protective effect against breast cancer, through decreasing the lifetime menstrual cycles, as researchers have highlighted that women who had breast cancer had more menstrual cycles before the first full-term pregnancy [24]. The first full-term pregnancy also stimulates a regular growth of breast cells resulting in fully mature breasts. Typically, breast cells before the first full-term pregnancy are very active and immature, therefore a delay in childbearing contributes significantly to increasing the rate of breast cancer prevalence [25]. Breast cancer incidence during pregnancy is about 2–3% of total cases of breast cancer [26]. However, diagnosis and treatment of pregnant women with breast cancer is a challenging issue, therefore it is essential that a woman with any breast lumps during pregnancy is referred to multidisciplinary professionals.

2.3.6 Race and ethnicity

The effects of race and ethnicity in shaping the disparities in breast cancer are persistently discussed in clinical investigations. Research studies have diagnosed breast cancer incidences while categorising their research population into local communities, migrant communities, Asians, Black people, White Europeans, etc. Studies have concluded with evidence that some populations are at higher risk of developing breast cancer in comparison to other female populations. Researchers have investigated various factors in relation to race and ethnicity and the incidence of breast cancer such as environmental, behavioural, biological factors, in addition to other factors including social and economic factors, etc [27–29].

2.3.7 Breast composition (density)

Dense breast tissue is not abnormal, and it is very common for women to have dense breasts. However, dense breast tissue is one of the factors that put women at higher risk of getting breast cancer and possibly four to six times more likely to get the disease. Dense breasts are not related to the size of the breast, it cannot be self-examined, and it can make it harder to read mammography results compared to women with fatty breasts. However, on a mammogram a way to measure the breast density is by measuring the thickness of the breast tissue [30]. A dense breast has less fatty tissue but more fibrous and glandular tissue, and on a mammogram, fat appears dark, while breast gland tissue looks light. Similar to gland tissue, breast tumours and calcifications look light on a mammogram, and this can make cancers difficult to be seen as it can merge inside the breast tissue [30]. Therefore, other modalities such as ultrasound imaging are used to aid mammography in screening patients with dense breasts. Breast density assessment is included in the Breast Imaging Reporting and Database Systems (BI-RADS), and it is classified into four categories; (A) mostly fatty breast tissue, (B) scattered fibroglandular breast tissue, (C) heterogeneously dense breast tissue and (D) extremely dense breast tissue [31]. Breast density can also be passed down from mothers with dense breasts to their daughters who are also expected to have dense breasts; however, other factors can influence breast composition [32].

2.3.8 Drinking alcohol and its effect on breast cancer

Likewise, the use of alcohol is not only associated with the occurrence of breast cancer the first time but also associated with the recurrence of breast cancer in breast cancer patients. Women drinking alcohol have a higher risk of getting breast cancer and the risk is increased by 50% in women who drink excessively (about 45 g/day of alcohol) [5, 33]. The mechanism behind this is believed to be associated with the effect of alcohol on the levels of circulating oestrogen [11]. Drinking alcohol may also put women at a higher risk of developing breast cancer through causing damage to DNA in cells [34].

References

[1] Siegel R, Miller K and Jemal A 2016 Cancer statistics, 2016 *CA: Cancer J. Clin.* **66** 7–30

[2] Solomon E 2016 *Introduction to Human Anatomy and Physiology* (Missouri: Elsevier)

[3] Michell M 2010 *Breast Cancer* (New York: Cambridge University Press)

[4] American Cancer Society 2018 *What is breast cancer?* (American Cancer Society) (https://cancer.org/cancer/breast-cancer/about/what-is-breast-cancer.html). Accessed 2018

[5] Veronesi U, Goldhirsch A, Veronesi P, Gentilini O and Leonardi M 2017 *Breast Cancer: Innovations in Research and Management* (Cham: Springer)

[6] Taghian A and Halyard M 2012 *Breast Cancer* (New York: Demos Medical Publishing)

[7] breastcancer.org 2018 *Breast cancer stages* (breastcancer.org) (https://breastcancer.org/symptoms/diagnosis/staging). Accessed 2020

[8] cancerresearchuk.org 2018 *Breast cancer statistics* (cancerresearchuk.org) (https://cancerresearchuk.org/health-professional/cancer-statistics/statistics-by-cancer-type/breast-cancer#-heading-Zero). Accessed 2022

[9] Fan L, Goss P and Strasser-Weippl K 2015 Current status and future projections of breast cancer in Asia *Breast Care* 372–8 2015

[10] Peng L, Xu T, Long T and Zuo H 2016 Association between BRCA status and P53 status in breast cancer: a meta-analysis *Med. Sci. Monit.* **2016** 1939–45

[11] Wyld L, Markopoulos C, Leidenius M and Senkus-Konefka E 2018 *Breast Cancer Management for Surgeons: A European Multidisciplinary Textbook* (Cham: Springer)

[12] breastcancer.org 2018 *Age* (breastcancer.org) (https://breastcancer.org/risk/factors/age). Accessed 2018

[13] CDC GOV 2021 *Breast cancer* (CDC GOV) (https://cdc.gov/cancer/breast/basic_info/risk_-factors.htm). Accessed 2021

[14] breastcancer.org 2018 *Genetics* (breastcancer.org) (https://breastcancer.org/risk/factors/genetics). Accessed 2018

[15] Hanenberg H and Andreassen P 2018 PALB2 (partner and localizer of BRCA2) *Atlas Genet. Cytogenet. Oncol. Haematol.* **22** 484–90

[16] Rainville I, Hatcher S, Rosenthal E, Larson K, Bernhisel R, Meek S, Gorringe H, Mundt E and Manley S 2020 High risk of breast cancer in women with biallelic pathogenic variants in CHEK2 *Breast Cancer Res. Treat.* **180** 503–9

[17] NHS UK 2018 *Predictive genetic tests for cancer risk genes* (NHS UK) (https://nhs.uk/conditions/predictive-genetic-tests-cancer/). Accessed 2020

[18] Mørch L, Skovlund C, Hannaford P, Iversen L, Fielding S and Lidegaard Ø 2017 Contemporary hormonal contraception and the risk of breast cancer *New Engl. J. Med.* **2017** 2228–39

[19] Beaber E, Buist D, Barlow W, Malone K, Reed S and Li C 2014 Recent oral contraceptive use by formulation and breast cancer risk among women 20 to 49 years of age *Cancer Res.* **74** 4078–89

[20] NHS UK 2015 *Menopause treatment* (NHS UK) (https://nhs.uk/conditions/menopause/treatment/). Accessed 2018

[21] Narod S 2011 Hormone replacement therapy and the risk of breast cancer *Nat. Rev. Clin. Oncol.* **8** 669–76

[22] Beral V, Reeves G, Bull D and Green J 2011 Breast cancer risk in relation to the interval between menopause and starting hormone therapy *J. Natl. Cancer Inst.* **103** 296–305

[23] Husby A, Wohlfahrt J, Øyen N and Melbye M 2018 Pregnancy duration and breast cancer risk *Nat. Commun.* **2018** 4255

[24] Olsson H and Olsson M 2020 The menstrual cycle and risk of breast cancer: a review *Front. Oncol.* **10** 21

[25] breastcancer.org 2021 *Pregnancy history* (breastcancer.org) (https://breastcancer.org/risk/factors/pregnancy_hist). Accessed 2021

[26] Heller S and Moy L 2017 *Breast Oncology: Techniques, Indications, and Interpretation* (Cham: Springer)

[27] Daly B and Olopade O 2015 Race, ethnicity, and the diagnosis of breast cancer *JAMA* **313** 141–2

[28] Chlebowski R *et al* 2005 Ethnicity and breast cancer: factors influencing differences in incidence and outcome *J. Natl. Cancer Inst.* **97** 439–48

[29] Gathani T, Ali R, Balkwill A, Green J, Reeves G, Beral V and Moser K 2014 Ethnic differences in breast cancer incidence in England are due to differences in known risk factors for the disease: prospective study *Br. J. Cancer* **110** 224–9 On behalf of the Million Women Study Collaborators

[30] breastcancer.org 2018 *Dense breasts* (breastcancer.org) (https://breastcancer.org/risk/factors/dense_breasts). Accessed 2018

[31] Shetty M 2015 *Breast Cancer Screening and Diagnosis: A Synopsis* (New York: Springer)

[32] cancer.gov 2020 *Dense breasts: Answers to commonly asked questions* (cancer.gov) (https://cancer.gov/types/breast/breast-changes/dense-breasts). Accessed 2020

[33] Seitz H, Pelucchi C, Bagnardi V and La Vecchia C 2012 Epidemiology and pathophysiology of alcohol and breast cancer: update 2012 *Alcohol Alcoholism* **47** 204–12

[34] breastcancer.org 2018 *Drinking alcohol* (breastcancer.org) (https://breastcancer.org/risk/factors/alcohol). Accessed 2018

IOP Publishing

Breast Cancer and Medical Imaging

Mohammed Erkhawan Hameed Rasheed and Mansour Youseffi

Chapter 3

Breast cancer prevention and breast cancer types

Chapter 3 presents a review of the existing breast cancer prevention strategies and the control of the disease. The common prevention strategies to deal with breast cancer are associated with the existing as well as new emerging risk factors, including modification of lifestyle and eating habits, and prevention through having early pregnancy and breast feeding. Other prevention strategies include taking medicines as well as prevention through surgery. This chapter also discusses the symptoms of breast cancer and the various types of the disease. Likewise, the chapter discusses the prevalence of breast cancer in young women in addition to pregnancy-associated breast cancers as well as the incidence of breast cancer in men.

3.1 Breast cancer prevention

Based on the range of identified risk factors associated with breast cancer, clinical investigators have highlighted the different types of prevention strategies for dealing with the above-mentioned risk factors. Women with a higher risk of breast cancer may benefit from the prevention strategies and treatments that are available to lower the risks of getting the disease. Although different strategies have been developed in the past, considering the primary and secondary preventions in addition to the choices and applicability of an effective breast cancer prevention strategy are dependent on the severity of the disease and the conditions of each case. These preventions are discussed precisely, while keeping focus on the factors that need to be considered to prevent the occurrence of breast cancer the first time as well as to avoid the prevalence of subsequent breast cancer [1, 2].

3.1.1 Modification of lifestyle and eating habits

Changing lifestyle and diet is recognised as a recommended prevention strategy to lower the risks of breast cancer in women with a higher risk of developing breast cancer. For all women, regular exercise and maintaining a healthy body weight is recommended as a dedicated cancer prevention effort. Clinical investigations have presented evidence that eating fruit and vegetables as well as a balanced diet may lower breast cancer risks [1].

The effect of a Mediterranean diet has also been investigated for cancer prevention, including the significant components of the diet such as a balanced ratio of omega 6 and omega 3, fibre and fatty acids in addition to antioxidants and polyphenols [2]. Similarly, other studies have established the efficiency of a diet based on Mediterranean and wholegrain recipes and philosophies connected with modest physical activities in contributing towards the incidence of additional breast cancer events in women already experiencing breast cancer. Researchers have highlighted that by increasing awareness among women, including those affected with breast cancer, about the common meals and exercise sessions associated with a healthy lifestyle, the risk of breast cancer can ultimately be reduced by as much as a third [3, 4].

3.1.2 Early pregnancy and breast feeding

A protective factor for breast cancer is to reduce the exposure of breast tissue to oestrogen. During pregnancy oestrogen levels are lower, therefore women have a lower risk of getting breast cancer if they had a full-term pregnancy before the age of 30 years. Likewise, breast feeding may keep oestrogen levels lower as well. Women who breast-feed for a full year or more have a lower risk of breast cancer [5]. Therefore, having children earlier rather than later and breast feeding are recommended options for women to lower their breast cancer risk.

3.1.3 Taking medicines

One of the most common breast cancer prevention strategies is using pharmaceutical drugs and medicines. Evidence from clinical investigations has revealed that tamoxifen and raloxifene (known as selective oestrogen receptor modulators (SERMs)) and anastrozole and exemestane (known as aromatase inhibitors (AIs)) can be used to reduce the risk of breast cancer. However, these medications act only to reduce the risk of a specific breast cancer type called oestrogen receptor-positive ((ER)-positive) breast cancer, which accounts for about two-thirds of all cases of breast cancer. Tamoxifen's common side effects include vaginal discharge, night sweats, hot flashes and blood clots, while the side effects of raloxifene include joint and muscle pain, weight gain, vaginal dryness and hot flashes. The aromatase inhibitors' common side effects include vaginal dryness, hot flashes, fatigue, joint and muscle pain, and headaches [6].

Contrary to the effectiveness of such pharmaceutical drugs in reducing the risk of breast cancer, researchers have also acknowledged the risks associated with the consumption of these medicines, as they are not well tolerated by women. Academic investigators have further highlighted that poor adherence to these medications and clinical trials that do not look at the impact on the quality of life of breast cancer patients ultimately raise questions regarding the effectiveness of pharmaceutical-based treatments [7]. It is crucial to evaluate the consequences and effects of using these medications in order to reduce the risk of breast cancer according to the aforementioned associated risk factors.

From examination of the different prevention strategies available across the globe to prevent the risk of breast cancer, it was found that the effectiveness and feasibility of these pharmaceutical prevention strategies vary case-by-case and therefore they cannot be implemented in a generalised and standard way. There is a possibility that women suffering from advanced stages of breast cancer cannot be treated with pharmaceuticals. In such situations, surgery is mainly the considerable prevention strategy for women.

3.1.4 Prevention through surgery

Breast-conserving surgery (BCS) with or without irradiation is also suggested for breast cancer prevention among women diagnosed with early breast cancer. Surgery is helpful in removing the affected areas and tissues permanently. Clinical investigators have confirmed the role of risk-reducing surgery especially in hereditary breast cancer cases [8]. Breast-conserving surgery is also known as lumpectomy, segmental mastectomy, partial mastectomy or quadrantectomy, and it is a type of surgery initiated to remove cancer and to leave as much healthy breast tissue as possible in the body. At present, BCS is the benchmark treatment for patients with stages 0, I and II invasive breast cancers [9].

Other types of prevention surgeries include mastectomy and breast reconstruction. Mastectomy is defined as a preventive strategy to avoid the transfer of breast cancer to other areas of the body. Mastectomy consists of the removal of the whole breast and is mainly suggested to patients suffering from a large and widely spread breast cancer or patients suffering from more than one cancer in the breast [10, 11]. In rare cases, clinicians also suggest double mastectomy. Evidence further suggests that patients experiencing mastectomy also prefer going through breast reconstruction surgeries such as implant reconstruction and flap reconstruction. Breast cancer surgery is considered to be a significant choice for patients when they are not left with any other options [12].

3.2 Breast cancer control

Prevention, early detection, diagnosis and treatment, rehabilitation and palliative care are the main steps involved in breast cancer control. Prevention of breast cancer is mostly connected to the control of risk factors leading to the diseases. It is important to highlight that breast cancer is a non-communicable disease and therefore integrated care and control can result in highly effective and long-term outcomes for patients. Usually, healthcare regulatory bodies participate in increasing public awareness about the need to adopt a lifestyle capable of modifying the risk factors. However, despite the adoption of risk-reducing measures to achieve the goal of prevention, the effectiveness and feasibility of these prevention strategies vary on a case-by-case basis and therefore this cannot be implemented in a generalised and standard way. There is a possibility that women suffering from advanced stages of breast cancer cannot be treated with pharmaceuticals and modification of diet and lifestyle. In such situations, surgery is the only considerable prevention strategy [13].

3.3 Breast cancer symptoms

Similar to the categorisation of breast cancer into different stages and types, clinical investigators have also segmented the symptoms of breast cancer according to invasiveness and non-invasiveness. Occurrence and mortality rates linked to invasive breast cancer are quite high across the globe, where thousands of women die from the disease. A range of symptoms have been identified with invasive breast cancer including the presence of a mass or lump in the breast. A lump is more likely to be cancer when it is painless, hard and has uneven edges. Any unusual changes, like the following in the breast, may be a symptom of breast cancer: swelling of all or part of the breast, skin dimpling or irritation, nipple and breast pain, nipple retraction, changing appearance of the nipple or breast skin resulting in redness, rash or thickening, any nipple bleeding or discharge other than breast milk [14]. Significant importance is given to invasive breast cancer due to its potential to spread to other parts of the body. Identification of the right symptom is essential for the identification of the correct breast cancer type.

3.4 Breast cancer types

There are many different breast cancer types, and they may start in various areas of the breast. Each breast cancer type depends on the specific breast cells that are affected, and they are named on the basis of where they form and how far they have spread. There are common breast cancer types, such as ductal carcinoma *in situ*, and less common breast cancer types, such as Paget's disease of the nipple. *In situ* (non-invasive), invasive (infiltrating) and metastatic are the terms used to describe the extent of the breast cancer. In some breast cancers one breast tumour can be a combination of more than one type and sometimes the breast cancer cells may not form a tumour or lump in any way. The most widespread types of breast cancers are carcinomas.

3.4.1 Ductal carcinoma *in situ* (DCIS)

Ductal carcinoma *in situ*, which is also known as intraductal carcinoma, refers to the incidence of breast cancer when the cancer cells are found inside the ducts of the breast. DCIS is a non-invasive or pre-invasive breast cancer, i.e., cancer has not completely developed or spread into the surrounding areas. DCIS is counted as stage 0 breast cancer. In general, DCIS has no symptoms or signs; however, a breast lump may be found sometimes in the breast or discharge from the nipple [15]. It should be noted that almost all females diagnosed with this early-stage breast cancer can be cured and the chances of a recurrence are less than 30%. However, the majority of recurrences occur within 5–10 years from the first diagnosis. Furthermore, DCIS accounts for approximately 20–25% of all newly detected cases of breast cancer in the United States [16].

3.4.2 Invasive ductal carcinoma (IDC)

Invasive ductal carcinoma, sometimes known as infiltrating ductal carcinoma, happens when the cancer cells have spread out to the ducts of the breast and started invading the tissues. IDC is an invasive breast cancer, meaning it can spread into lymph nodes and other parts of the body through the bloodstream and the lymphatic system. IDC initially may have no symptoms but often there is an abnormal area or a new mass or lump in the breast that turns up during a breast self-examination (BSE) or a mammogram screening. IDC is the most common breast cancer type, and it accounts for about 70–80% of all detected breast cancer cases. In the United States about 180 000 of women are diagnosed with IDC each year [17].

3.4.3 Lobular carcinoma *in situ* (LCIS)

Lobular carcinoma *in situ*, also called lobular neoplasia, is a non-invasive breast cancer, i.e., cancer is confined to the lobules of the breast and has not spread to the surrounding fatty tissue or other parts of the body. Women with LCIS have an increased risk of developing an invasive breast cancer later in life in the same or the other breast. In general, LCIS affects more than one lobule and usually there are no symptoms, as it does not cause a lump or changes that can be felt or seen on a mammogram [18]; therefore, women with LCIS need to take regular mammogram screening and clinical breast examinations. LCIS is typically counted as a risk factor for developing breast cancer, apart from one type of LCIS known as Pleomorphic Breast Cancer (Lobular), which may turn into invasive breast cancer; therefore, surgery is performed to totally remove it [19].

3.4.4 Invasive lobular carcinoma (ILC)

Invasive lobular carcinoma or infiltrating lobular carcinoma is the second most common form of invasive breast cancer after IDC and it accounts for about 10% of all invasive breast cancers [20]. ILC starts initially in one of the lobules, i.e., the milk producing glands of the breast and then the cancer cells spread to other parts of the breast. ILC is usually found in both breasts, but it can also spread to the lymph nodes and other parts of the body. ILC tends to occur later in life from late 50s to early 60s. Like IDC, ILC at first may have no signs but sometimes an abnormal area in the breast turns up during a mammogram screening or there is a thickening in the breast that can be felt.

3.4.5 Inflammatory breast cancer (IBC)

Inflammatory breast cancer is identified as a rare type of breast cancer and it is known for being a very aggressive disease. IBC at diagnosis is either stage III or IV, depending on whether it has spread to the surrounding lymph nodes or to other tissues too. IBC in the United States accounts for about 1–5% of all cases of breast cancer. IBC grows and spreads very fast with symptoms getting worse within hours or days. The disease generally develops after the age of 50 and its indications vary from simple to more complex prognosis such as dermal lymphatic invasion.

IBC usually starts with the feeling of heaviness or thickness in the breast, and it tends to grow in the form of tissue layers. The cancer cells block the lymph vessels causing the breasts to become inflamed and swell. The symptoms may include breast swelling and redness, breasts having an orange-peel appearance, breasts feeling tender and achy, lymph nodes swelling, nipple inversion and nipple flattening [21].

3.4.6 Paget's disease of the nipple

Paget's disease of the nipple is a rare type of breast cancer; about 1–4% of breast cancer patients have Paget's disease of the nipple. It usually develops after the age of 50 and is recognised by changes that occur in the appearance of the nipple and areola. The symptoms of Paget's disease are itchy, red, scaly and irritated nipple and areola. The disease first starts from the ducts of the nipple and then spreads to the surface of the nipple and areola. Additionally, patients may notice thickening and scaling of the skin, flattering of the nipple and they may experience some bloody or yellowish discharge from the nipple. There is a strong relationship between DCIS and the prevalence of Paget's disease and, in most cases, the presence of Paget's disease is an indication of the presence of an early form of cancer. Paget's disease mainly affects one breast, and it is often mistaken for eczema, but eczema generally affects the areola not the nipple [22].

3.4.7 HER2-positive breast cancer

The HER2 (human epidermal growth factor receptor 2) gene is responsible for making HER2 proteins. These proteins are receptors located on the cells of the breast and they help in controlling healthy growth, division and self-repair of the breast cells. About 1 out of 5 women with breast cancer are HER2-positive [23]. The cancer cells of this type of breast cancer have more HER2 proteins and they cause the cancer cells to grow and spread very aggressively and more rapidly than the cells that have normal levels of HER2 proteins. HER2 gene amplification occurs when this gene does not work properly and it makes too many copies of itself. This huge number of HER2 genes inform the breast cells to make too many HER2 receptors, which in return causes the breast cells to grow and divide in a way that cannot be controlled. The growth of this type of cancer is relatively faster than the other types of breast cancer. As far as the symptoms of the HER2 breast cancer are concerned, they are like the other types of breast cancer symptoms. The treatment of both early and metastatic HER2-positive breast cancer using anti-HER2 treatment has changed this type of cancer's natural biology and it has further helped in increasing the survival rates of almost 5 years in patients with metastatic HER2-positive breast cancer. The effective interventions have ultimately led towards a pathological complete response by 75% of patients [24].

3.5 Prevalence of breast cancer in young women

Young women are considered as one of the most vulnerable population groups affected by breast cancer. About 6.6% of the cases of breast cancer are diagnosed in women under 40 years old [25, 26]. Age is an independent prognostic factor, indicating that young women experience more aggressive subtypes of breast cancer such as triple-negative or HER2-positive breast cancers. It is also important to highlight that young women are subjected to experience advanced stages of breast cancer due to different factors such as delayed diagnosis. Consequently, such breast cancer cases perhaps transformed into local or regional recurrences and distant metastases. Regardless of the independence of the age factor, the prevailing breast cancer found in young women can further be categorised differently in different parts of the world such as in Europe, North America, Africa, Asia and other countries. In a similar context, investigations on the prevalence of breast cancer rates in young women from selected countries such as Italy 0.6%, France 0.59%, UK 0.5%, Lebanon 0.45% and USA 0.45% identified these as the top five countries with a higher cumulative risk [25].

Among the most influential factors affecting the prevailing breast cancer in young women include the long-term use of oral contraceptives, body mass index and a high consumption of animal fat. Findings have also highlighted that obesity is associated with both pre- and postmenopausal breast cancer risks. Despite their influence on the incidence of breast cancer, studies have highlighted that these factors are modifiable relative to the set of non-modifiable factors such as family history and gene mutations. Similarly, the significance of adverse pathological factors cannot be undermined [27]. Furthermore, survival rates in the younger women are shown to be worse in comparison to older women [28, 29].

3.6 Breast cancer and pregnancy

Pregnancy-associated breast cancers are also identified as highly critical in the younger population. Young pregnant women with oestrogen receptor-negative tumours and high-grade tumours are expected to have a lower prognosis [30]. Evidence has suggested that it may be difficult to diagnose breast cancer in pregnant or lactating women and, in the case of the presence of a breast lump during pregnancy, the case is referred to multidisciplinary professionals [29]. Studies have further shown that diagnosis and treatment of pregnant young women with breast cancer becomes a challenging issue for the clinicians because several effective imaging techniques such as bone scanning, pelvic X-ray and computed tomography scan, and treatment procedures cannot be applied. Pregnancy-associated breast cancers are every so often misunderstood as only those which are diagnosed during the pregnancy term of nine months, whereas this also includes breast cancers diagnosed in the first postpartum year. Investigators have suggested that a delay in childbearing is contributing significantly to increasing breast cancer in young women [31]. In general, clinical professionals decide upon the therapeutic strategies for determining the tumour biology, tumour stage, gestational age and other socio-demographic factors affecting decisions regarding each case.

3.7 Breast cancer in men

Additionally, for a better understanding of breast cancer incidences in the female population, analysis of male breast cancer is also significant. Statistics have shown that male breast cancer is very rare and only less than 1% of all breast cancer types is likely to develop in men [32]. Researchers have highlighted the risk factors, biology, diagnosis, treatment and survivorship of breast cancer in men. Researchers have indicated that the most considerable risk factors responsible for breast cancer in men include BRCA2 mutations, age, circumstances capable of modifying the oestrogen/androgen ratio, in addition to radiation [33].

Symptoms of breast cancer in men include a breast lump, swollen glands in the armpit, inverted nipple, sore nipple and nipple discharge [34]. Researchers have further highlighted that the differences in the disease biology in men do not affect the diagnostic approaches and treatments chosen to deal with the cases, meaning that both males as well as females are diagnosed with employment of the same diagnostic approaches and treatments, one of the reasons behind which is the lack of research in male patients [33]. Researchers have highlighted that breast cancer in males is subjected to survival issues associated with the sexual and hormonal side effects associated with endocrine therapies. The variations in the rates of cancer among men are linked with variations in behavioural risk factors as well as using screening services in addition to being exposed to infections that are cancer-causing. Researchers have also highlighted the strategies used to control cancer, such as using vaccinations, screening programmes, exercises and controlling body weight in addition to controlling smoking and drinking alcohol [35].

References

[1] Colditz G and Bohlke K 2014 Priorities for the primary prevention of breast cancer *CA: Cancer J. Clin.* **64** 186–94

[2] Giacosa A *et al* 2013 Cancer prevention in Europe: the Mediterranean diet as a protective choice *Eur. J. Cancer Prev.* **22** 90–5

[3] Villarini A *et al* 2012 Lifestyle and breast cancer recurrences: the DIANA-5 trial *Tumori J.* **98** 1–18

[4] NHS UK 2016 *Prevention* (NHS UK) (https://nhs.uk/conditions/breast-cancer/prevention/). Accessed 2018

[5] breastcancer.org 2018 *Breastfeeding history* (breastcancer.org) (https://breastcancer.org/risk/factors/breastfeed_hist). Accessed 2018

[6] Pluchinotta A 2015 *The Outpatient Breast Clinic: Aiming at Best Practice* (New York: Springer)

[7] Liekweg A, Westfeld M, Braun M, Zivanovic O, Schink T, Kuhn W and Jaehde U 2012 Pharmaceutical care for patients with breast and ovarian cancer *Support Care Cancer* **20** 2669–77

[8] Kunkler I, Williams L, Jack W, Cameron D and Dixon J 2015 Breast-conserving surgery with or without irradiation in women aged 65 years or older with early breast cancer (PRIME II): a randomised controlled trial *Lancet Oncol.* **16** 266–73

[9] Brunicardi F, Anderson D, Billiar T, Dunn D, Hunter H, Pollock R and Matthews J 2014 *Schwartz's Current Practice of General Surgery (EBOOK)* (New York: McGraw Hill Professional)

[10] Veronesi U, Goldhirsch A, Veronesi P, Gentilini O and Leonardi M 2017 *Breast Cancer: Innovations in Research and Management* (Cham: Springer)

[11] Washington C and Leaver D 2015 *Principles and Practice of Radiation Therapy—E-Book* (Missouri: Elsevier)

[12] bcna.org.au 2021 *Types of surgery* (bcna.org.au) (https://bcna.org.au/understanding-breast-cancer/treatment/surgery/types-of-surgery/). Accessed 2021

[13] WHO 2018 *Breast Cancer Control* (WHO). (http://who.int/cancer/detection/breastcancer/en/index3.html). Accessed 2018

[14] cancer.org 2018 *Breast cancer signs and symptoms* (cancer.org). (https://cancer.org/cancer/breast-cancer/about/breast-cancer-signs-and-symptoms.html). Accessed 30 May 2018

[15] Newman L A and Bensenhaver J M 2015 *Ductal Carcinoma* In Situ *and Microinvasive/ Borderline Breast Cancer* (New York: Springer)

[16] Kanbayashi C and Iwata H 2017 Current approach and future perspective for ductal carcinoma *in situ* of the breast *Jpn. J. Clin. Oncol.* **47** 671–7

[17] breastcancer.org 2018 *Invasive Ductal Carcinoma (IDC)* (breastcancer.org). (https://breast-cancer.org/symptoms/types/idc). Accessed 2018

[18] Peart O 2018 *LANGE Q&A: Mammography Examination* 4th edn (New York: McGraw Hill Education)

[19] American Cancer Society 2016 *Does LCIS need to be treated?* (American Cancer Society). (https://cancer.org/cancer/breast-cancer/treatment/treatment-of-breast-cancer-by-stage/treat-ment-of-lobular-carcinoma-in *situ*-lcis.html). Accessed 2018

[20] Selvi R 2015 *Breast Diseases: Imaging and Clinical Management* (New Delhi: Springer)

[21] National Cancer Institute 2016 *Inflammatory breast cancer* (National Institutes of Health) (https://cancer.gov/types/breast/ibc-fact-sheet). Accessed 2018

[22] NHS UK 2016 *Paget's disease of the nipple* (NHS UK). (https://nhs.uk/conditions/pagets-disease-nipple/). Accessed 2018

[23] American Cancer Society 2018 *Targeted therapy for breast cancer* (American Cancer Society). (https://cancer.org/cancer/breast-cancer/treatment/targeted-therapy-for-breast-can-cer.html). Accessed 2018

[24] Loibl S and Gianni L 2017 HER2-positive breast cancer *Lancet* **389** 2415–29

[25] Assi H, Khoury K, Dbouk H, Khalil L, Mouhieddine T and Saghir N 2013 Epidemiology and prognosis of breast cancer in young women *J. Thoracic Dis.* 2–8 2013

[26] Zhang X, Yang J, Cai H and Ye Y 2018 Young age is an independent adverse prognostic factor in early stage breast cancer: a population-based study *Cancer Manag. Res.* 4005–18 2018

[27] Caldarella A, Crocetti E, Bianchi S, Vezzosi V, Urso C, Biancalani M and Zappa M 2011 Female breast cancer status according to ER, PR and HER2 expression: a population based analysis *Pathol. Oncol. Res.* **17** 753–8

[28] Anders C, Johnson R, Litton J, Phillips M and Bleyere A 2009 Breast cancer before age 40 years *Semin. Oncol.* **36** 237–49

[29] RCOG 2011 *Pregnancy and Breast Cancer Green-Top Guideline No. 12* (Royal College of Obstetricians and Gynaecologists)

[30] Keyser E, Staat B, Fausett M and Shields A 2012 Pregnancy-associated breast cancer *Rev. Obstetr. Gynecol.* **5** 94–9

[31] Floris G, Han S and Amant F 2014 Pregnancy-associated breast cancer *J. Pediatr. Neonatal Individ. Med. (JPNIM)* **3** 94

[32] Papadakis M, McPhee S and Rabow M 2015 *Current Medical Diagnosis and Treatment 2016* (New York: McGraw-Hill Education)

[33] Ruddy K and Winer E 2013 Male breast cancer: risk factors, biology, diagnosis, treatment, and survivorship *Annal. Oncol.* **24** 1434–43

[34] NHS UK 2017 *Breast cancer in men* (NHS UK) (https://nhs.uk/conditions/breast-cancer-in-men/). Accessed 2018

[35] Torre L, Sauer A, Chen M, Kagawa-Singer M, Jemal A and Siegel R 2016 Cancer statistics for Asian Americans, Native Hawaiians, and Pacific Islanders, 2016: converging incidence in males and females *CA: Cancer J. Clin.* **66** 182–202

IOP Publishing

Breast Cancer and Medical Imaging

Mohammed Erkhawan Hameed Rasheed and Mansour Youseffi

Chapter 4

Breast cancer treatments

Chapter 4 discusses the various treatment choices that are available to treat breast cancer, depending on the type and stage of each case. The National Health Service (NHS) in the United Kingdom has highlighted a list of the main breast cancer treatments available including surgery, radiotherapy, chemotherapy, hormone therapy and biological therapy (targeted therapy) [1]. Surgery and radiotherapy treatments are local treatments, i.e., a tumour is treated with no damage to other body parts. On the other hand, chemotherapy, hormone therapy and biological therapy are systematic treatments, i.e., the drugs that are used to treat breast cancers can reach almost all parts of the body. Patients may get one or a combination of these treatments. Treatments offered are either for full recovery from the disease or in cases of patients with advanced stages of breast cancer, treatments are offered as pain relief and better quality of life. In most cases, it is upon the personal preferences of the patient as well as their close family members to choose among the different treatment options available. However, the chosen option needs to be compatible with the type of breast cancer, stage of the disease, patient's age as well as their overall health. In general, a multidisciplinary team (MDT) is appointed to provide care and treatment. A MDT is a team of healthcare professionals and specialists who work together for each cancer type [1]. This chapter also discusses a range of complementary and alternative medicine (CAM) used for cancer patients in various parts of the world including traditional Chinese medicine (TCM). It should be noted that some sections from this chapter about CAM were presented at the 11th International Conference on Mathematical Modeling in Physical Sciences (2022) and submitted as a conference paper for publication in the American Institute of Physics (AIP) Conference Proceedings [2].

4.1 Surgery

Surgery is one of the most common types of breast cancer treatments and it is the first treatment that patients usually undergo as their primary treatment modality [3].

There are different types of surgical options available including breast-conserving surgery (lumpectomy) and total removal of the breast (mastectomy), all depending on the severity of the condition. Breast-conserving surgery (BCS) is the surgery of removing the tumour from the breast while leaving as much healthy breast tissue as possible. BCS is typically chosen for women with early-stage breast cancers, but in most cases, patients will also get radiotherapy treatment. During the surgery, the tumour is removed along with a rim of healthy tissue around it, called the margin of resection or the surgical margin, to make sure that all the cancer cells have been removed. The presentation of a precise assessment of resection margins is an important part of a successful local treatment of breast cancer. Likewise, mastectomy is the surgery of removing the entire breast, including all the breast tissue and other nearby healthy tissue and lymph nodes, depending on each patient's specific situation. Mastectomy is either unilateral, i.e., one breast is surgically removed, or some patients may get a double (bilateral) mastectomy, which is a risk-reducing surgery in which both breasts are removed [1]. The side effects associated with the different types of breast cancer surgeries may include discomfort, pain, drowsiness, fatigue, seroma (swelling in the breast or armpit) infection and other problems in the general health of the patient. Patients with surgery to the armpit may get more discomfort and pain and other complications including dysfunction of the upper limb related to surgeries such as axillary lymph node dissection (ALND) and sentinel lymph node biopsy (SLNB). To deal with such side effects associated with these breast cancer surgeries, patients are recommended to go for post-operative physical therapy and post-surgery exercises such as strength and resistance exercises, concentrating on pain and discomfort management [4]. The quality of life (QOL) after breast cancer surgery may also become affected. QOL is usually better in patients following BCS compared to mastectomy. QOL includes social, emotional role functioning, fatigue symptoms, body image, arm symptoms and pain [5].

4.2 Chemotherapy

Chemotherapy or chemo is another type of treatment for breast cancer, which involves the use of cytotoxic medication to kill the cancer cells including any cancer cells that have spread to other body parts by metastasis. Anti-cancer drugs are given to patients intravenously through a drip directly into the blood and in some cases tablets are given as well. Breast cancer patients usually get chemotherapy after surgery to destroy any remaining cancer cells. When chemotherapy is given after surgery it is known as adjuvant chemotherapy and when it is given before surgery to reduce the size of the tumour so that it could be removed more easily, it is called neoadjuvant chemotherapy [6]. Different anti-cancer drugs are used for chemotherapy and in many cases a combination of three drugs is given at once. The choice of drugs and combinations depend on the type and severity of the breast cancer, and the treatment length is dependent on how well the chemotherapy is working and how well the patient can keep up with it along with the side effects they have. The main side effects of chemotherapy include anaemia, infection, fatigue, loss of appetite, vomiting, diarrhoea, hair changes and sore mouth and throat. Breast cancer survivors may also get long-term side effects such as impact on fertility, treatment-induced menopause, cardiovascular toxicity and cognitive impairment [1].

4.3 Radiotherapy (RT)

The other important treatment choice for breast cancer patients is radiation therapy (RT). RT uses doses of ionising radiation to kill or control the breast cancer cells. Radiotherapy may be offered on its own or in conjunction with surgery or chemotherapy. RT can be used after mastectomy or as a part of breast-conserving surgery to kill any remaining cancer cells around the affected area of the breast, or after mastectomy to minimise the local-regional recurrence risks and to improve long-term breast cancer-specific and overall survival. Radiotherapy is recommended after the patient has recovered from the surgical process and is open to different options including breast radiotherapy (which is offered after BCS, in which radio-therapy is delivered to all the remaining breast tissue), chest wall radiotherapy (which is delivered after mastectomy, in which radiation is applied to the chest wall), breast boost (in which a boost of high-dose radiation is applied to the affected area of the breast after surgery) and radiotherapy to the lymph nodes (in which radiation is applied to the armpit and the surrounding area of axilla to kill any cancer cells in the lymph nodes). Similar to surgery and chemotherapy, RT is also subject to side effects including skin reactions such as darkening and irritation, pain, fatigue and tiredness, armpit and chest hair loss, breast oedema and lymphoedema [1]. Likewise, modern techniques of radiotherapy such as deep inspiration breath hold (DIBH) are used for breast cancer treatment. Due to the position of the heart in the chest, which is slightly left of the centre, the DIBH technique is used in patients with left-sided breast cancer. In DIBH the patient takes a deep breath during radiotherapy and holds their breath at the same time as the radiation is delivered. DIBH is necessary to avoid the patient's heart from receiving any radiation dose.

4.4 Hormone treatment

Breast cancers that are stimulated by the hormones oestrogen or progesterone are called hormone receptor-positive (ER+) breast cancers. Hormone treatment works by lowering the amount of these hormones in the body or by blocking their action. Hormone therapy is either offered before surgery (called primary or neoadjuvant treatment) to reduce the size of the tumour to make it easier to be removed or it can be given after surgery (called adjuvant treatment) to reduce the risk of breast cancer coming back. Hormone treatment may also be offered as the only breast cancer treatment in patients who have other illnesses such as lung or heart illnesses and if their general health prevents them from having these treatments. However, the effectiveness of hormone treatment is dependent on the stage, age and the sensitiveness of the breast cancer to the hormones. In cases of an absence of any sensitivity, hormone treatment will have no effect. Tamoxifen, aromatase inhibitors and ovarian ablation or suppression are the main types of medicines used in hormonal therapy. The side effects of hormone therapy are mainly menopausal symptoms such as hot flushes and sweats, vaginal dryness, and psychological problems such as depressions and mood swings as well as loss of libido or sex drive. Other side effects include nausea, headaches, stiffness, joint pain and fatigue or tiredness [1].

4.5 Biological therapy (targeted therapy)

Biological therapy works by targeting the changes that occur in the cancer cells. The drugs used stop the growth and spread of the cancer cells. Unlike chemotherapy, targeted therapy drugs attack only the cancer cells and sometimes they may work better than chemotherapy. Targeted therapy is the treatment for breast cancers that are HER2-positive [7]. HER2-positive breast cancer has more HER2 proteins, and they make the cancer cells grow and spread faster than cancer cells with normal levels of HER2 proteins. Biological therapy using medications such as Trastuzumab (Herceptin) and Pertuzumab (Perjeta) are monoclonal antibodies used for the treatment of both early and metastatic HER2-positive breast cancer and they have changed this type of cancer's natural biology and further helped in increasing the survival rates of almost 5 years in patients with metastatic HER2-positive breast cancer. The effective interventions have ultimately led towards a pathological complete response by 75% of patients. The side effects of biological therapy are often mild such as pains, tiredness, fever, nausea and diarrhoea, but some side effects can be serious heart problems [8]. Likewise, breast cancer immunotherapy is part of biologic therapy, and it uses the patient's immune system as a treatment for breast cancer. Breast cancer immunotherapy is a type of systemic treatment used for breast cancer and is developing rapidly as several studies recently have demonstrated improved outcomes in treating some types of breast cancer. Immune Checkpoint Blockade (ICB) is the most investigated form of breast cancer immunotherapy. ICB is used as monotherapy or in combination with chemotherapy to improve treatment responses. Immunotherapy has shown helpful results for some patients, but it may cause severe side effects. Therefore, more research needs to be done to make advances in breast cancer treatment. The U.S. Food and Drug Administration (FDA) have approved several immunotherapy medicines to treat breast cancer such as Atezolizumab (Tecentriq) [9], which was granted accelerated approval. Tecentriq is used in combination with the chemotherapy drug Albumin-Bound Paclitaxel (Nab-paclitaxel or Abraxane) to treat triple-negative breast cancers. Triple-negative breast cancer is oestrogen receptor-negative, progesterone-receptor-negative and HER2-negative breast cancer. Triple-negative breast cancers are more aggressive than hormone receptor-positive or HER2-positive breast cancers [10].

4.6 Complementary and alternative medicine (CAM)

Complementary and alternative medicine (CAM) is either used to complement the standard cancer therapies given to cancer patients to help them cope with the symptoms and side effects and to improve their quality of life (QOL) such as the patient's emotional, social and physical wellbeing (including pain, that being the most important cause of distress among cancer patients), or to directly fight cancer as an alternative to conventional cancer treatments. The common practices of many complementary and alternative treatments emphasise good nutrition and prophy-laxis, and it is therefore believed that CAM works by boosting the natural immunity of the body to kill the cancer cells; however, more scientific research is needed to find out if the improvements in cancer patients' health are real and due to the complementary and alternative therapies used (i.e., not as a result of other treatments) and also to present scientific evidence that these treatments are safe to use and do not interact with conventional cancer therapies. The terms 'comple-mentary medicine' and 'alternative medicine' are often used together and usually in one sentence as: complementary and alternative medicine (CAM). However, complementary medicine, also known as integrative medicine, refers to treatments used side by side with standard cancer treatments of surgery, chemotherapy and radiotherapy. Complementary medicine is mainly used to help cancer patients feel better with the side effects and symptoms of conventional therapies. On the other hand, alternative medicine refers to nonstandard treatments being used instead of conventional medical therapies. Many different research studies have presented scientific evidence that CAM can encourage better overall health for cancer patients, it can strengthen the immune defences of the body, and aid cancer patients to manage the symptoms and side effects of the standard cancer treatments. In this section, clinically successful evidence regarding CAM treatments given to patients with cancer, including results of a number of medical research studies, is looked at to get a clearer idea on CAM used in different parts of the world to help people with cancer. The CAM treatments discussed in this work are a summary of the overall use of some CAM treatments against different types of cancers as supportive and palliative care especially in decreasing the side effects of conventional cancer therapies and to improve QOL. However, more research is needed on the topic of CAM so that it is effectively and safely used to treat and help people with cancer. Various CAM therapies are used worldwide to treat cancer including Cannabidiol (CBD), Zamzam Water (ZW), Graviola, Origanum Vulgare, Traditional Chinese Medicine (TCM) and Paris Polyphylla. Researchers have highlighted that comple-mentary medicines can help cancer patients feel better when used along with standard cancer treatments; for instance, CBD has proved beneficial for improving a variety of symptoms (such as pain and nausea) in cancer patients. Likewise, some alternative therapies such as TCM are approved to be used in China to treat various cancer tumours. Similarly, the side effects of conventional treatments and dissat-isfaction are also highlighted to be among the push factors to use CAM, while pull factors, on the other hand, included the positive aspects associated with CAM, such as the expectation of fewer side effects, stronger immunity and better QOL.

4.6.1 Cannabidiol

Cannabidiol (CBD) is a non-intoxicating chemical that comes from the cannabis sativa plant. Cannabidiol is a cannabinoid (CB) found in cannabis and it is non-psychoactive. Therefore, CBD has been used for pain relief and other tumour-associated symptoms with no mind-altering effects. CBD is one of many different cannabinoids and the two main cannabinoids, delta-9-tetrahydrocannabinol (d-9-THC) and cannabidiol [11, 12]. Cannabidiol is known to have a wide range of health benefits such as treating pain, anxiety, depression, epilepsy and has anti-inflammatory [13, 14] as well as anti-cancer activities [15]. CBD works by binding to the cannabinoid receptors such as cannabinoid receptor 1 (CB1) and cannabinoid receptor 2 (CB2) in the body and it can help in regulating the endocannabinoid system (ECS). The ECS is a molecular system that regulates and balances various processes in the body to maintain homeostasis such as helping the immune system identify when to attack and destroy foreign substances in the body in addition to other body processes including appetite, memory, metabolism, pain and sleep, etc [15, 16]. CBDs are used in cancer patients to kill cancer cells and prevent cancer cell migration and kill tumours [15]. CBDs have shown anti-tumour potentials and provided relief for tumour-associated symptoms as well as being active against oestrogen receptor-positive and oestrogen-resistant breast cancer cells. Furthermore, CBDs have been used to manage patients with advanced stages of breast cancer and to be effective in tumour progression deceleration in breast cancer patients at earlier stages.

4.6.2 Graviola (soursop)

Graviola, also known as soursop, is the fruit of a small evergreen tree that is broadleaf and flowering called Annona muricata. Annona muricata is found in the African and Latin American rainforests and is known for being used by people as an important source of food and medicine. Graviola has the flavour of a combination of apple and strawberry, and is usually used in making candy, juice and sorbet. Graviola is also known to have medicinal benefits such as treating viral and parasitic infections as well as arthritis and rheumatism [17, 18]. Graviola extracts can also help to treat other medical conditions such as slowing the spread of cancer and making conventional cancer treatments work better. Graviola is known for having anti-tumor and antioxidant properties and can help to treat cancer. Graviola extracts have shown anti-cancer effects and it can kill some types of cancer cells that are usually resistant to some drugs of chemotherapy [19, 20].

4.6.3 Origanum vulgare

Origanum vulgare or oregano is one of the herbs in the mint family Lamiaceae found in the Mediterranean, Eurasia and other parts of the world. Oregano is an invasive plant with a pink flower that has a potent flavour and is used in a variety of cuisines, and it is linked to health benefits. Oregano is known to have antibacterial properties, and it is effective against many organisms such as *Escherichia coli*, *Salmonella enterica* and *Clostridium difficile* [21]. Oregano oil is a natural anti-inflammatory herb. It has pain-relieving properties and is commonly used as a medication for cold sores, sore throats, nasal congestion, muscle pain and joint pain [22] and to reduce lower backache. Oregano is also high in antioxidants that help to prevent cell damage and cancer and also kill cancer cells. Oregano has shown anti-tumour effects in cancer models [23] and chemo preventive and therapeutic effects to modulate the growth and metastasis of cancer [24].

4.6.4 Zamzam water

Zamzam is the name of a well located in the sacred mosque in the city of Mecca, Saudi Arabia. The water that is taken from the well is known as Zamzam Water (ZW) and it is sacred to Muslims. ZW has a distinct taste, and it is colourless and odourless. ZW is rich in a variety of minerals, and it is naturally alkaline [25] with an average pH of 8.0 [26]. Studies have confirmed that ZW is pathogen-free causing no microbial growth [27] and also the quality and components of ZW have remained relatively unchanged for years [26]. ZW is consumed by many people on a daily basis especially in the cities of Mecca and Medina as a blessing and for its health benefits. According to Islamic sources, the prophet of Islam, Mohammed (peace be upon him) used to drink ZW and he used to say that ZW is a blessing, it is food that satisfies and a cure for the sick, and it is for whatever purpose for which it is drunk. In general, ZW may have cytotoxic effects [28] and may work as an anti-cancer agent to naturally treat cancer with no side effects [27, 29]. The right methodology of using ZW to treat cancer and other illnesses is simply by drinking it, and it is recommended when drinking ZW to pause to take a breath three times and then drink one's fill. ZW is absorbed by the stomach and the intestines and passed to the bloodstream to circulate all the way through the body in the form of body fluids. It is important to make sure that a genuine ZW is used, i.e., as it is obtained from the well in Mecca without changing it before use. If ZW is modified in any way, for example, if its pH is adjusted to a pH different than normal, it will have less effect on cancer cells [28]. Furthermore, ZW will totally lose its effectiveness when it is diluted and its pH is adjusted to a different pH than its normal pH, in addition to other changes. In a journal article published in 2019 [30], the authors showed that in their experiment, cancer cell growth was increased by ZW treatment and that ZW treatment suppressed the effect of chemotherapeutic agents, etc, and in the same paper, the authors stated that the methods they followed were 'ZW and DW were buffered using PBS and the pH was adjusted to 7.4. For the treatment, ZW and DW were diluted to 50% with RPMI medium (10% FBS)'. Therefore, when ZW is changed through dilution or pH change and other changes, then it is not ZW anymore but a different substance. And so, when a sample of ZW is used in a study that is a modified version of ZW, then the study is invalid, the results are simply inaccurate and therefore it cannot be claimed that ZW causes harm to cancer and that it interferes with chemotherapy. ZW is free from the holy mosques in Mecca and Medina under the management of the local governments. However, ZW is also sold in shops and sometimes online, and cannot be guaranteed to be a real sample of ZW; therefore, it is possible that ZW obtained from these sources is a modified version of ZW and so could be either contaminated or poisonous [31].

4.6.5 Traditional Chinese Medicine (TCM)

Traditional Chinese Medicine (TCM), including a variety of forms of herbal medicine, has been used for many years in China and other parts of the world for treating various health problems such as heart and circulatory diseases, mental health disorders (for example, depression and anxiety), in addition to respiratory diseases, etc. TCM is also approved in China to be used as alternative therapies to treat different types of cancer [32]. Chinese Herbal Medicine (CHM) is used to help reduce the side effects associated with chemotherapy, prevent cancer recurrence, enhance the body's immune system, as well as improving the QOL of cancer patients [33, 34]. The importance of CHM is in its effectiveness in treating tumours with minimum side effects and low toxicity [35, 36].

4.6.6 Paris polyphylla

Paris Polyphylla, also known as Multi-leaf Paris, is a flowering plant that grows up to 90 cm and produces flowers with green leaves that may reach up to 30 cm wide. Paris Polyphylla is a TCM herb that has a bitter taste, and its components are commonly used in China and other places in Asia to treat various forms of cancer and other illnesses such as infectious diseases and traumatic injuries [37]. Paris Polyphylla is known to have cytotoxic activities as well as antimicrobial, anti-cancer properties and it could reduce tumour growth [38–40].

4.7 Breast cancer recurrence

Breast cancer is recognised as one of the most life-threatening diseases as it can come back after treatment at any time, even decades after the occurrence and treatment of the original tumour. When breast cancer returns it is known as recurrence and it depends on whether it is a local recurrence (i.e., in the treated breasts) or a distant recurrence (i.e., in other parts of the body such as lymph nodes, bones, liver, lungs and brain) [3]. The incidence of breast cancer recurrence has various factors, such as the type of treatment, stressful life events, sociodemographic factors, and other physical and pathological factors. In discussing the psychological factors, along with the medical factors, it is necessary to investigate the prognostic association, such as severe life stressors, to identify the recurrence. Prevalence of breast cancer may also differ in young patients from older adult women. Gender-based differences are also considered significant in clinical investigations, indicating that the incidence of breast cancer can be different in the population of men and women. Clinical researchers have therefore highlighted that the recurrence of breast cancer should be considered on a case-by-case basis. However, improvements in systematic therapy have lowered breast cancer recurrence rates [3].

4.8 Blood marker test

Blood marker tests are used to predict breast cancer recurrence after treatment. However, blood marker tests are also performed before treatment to determine if cancer has spread to other parts of the body. Furthermore, blood marker tests performed during treatment are used to find out if the disease is responding to treatments. The CA125 marker test can be used to indicate the recurrence of breast cancer, while the CEA (carcinoembryonic antigen) marker test can be used to find out if breast cancer has spread to other parts of the body (metastasis). Moreover, a circulating tumour cells marker test may be used to signal that breast cancer is growing into the bloodstream, when there is high circulating tumour cell counts [41].

References

[1] NHS UK 2016 *Treatment* (NHS UK) (https://nhs.uk/conditions/breast-cancer/treatment/) Accessed 2018

[2] Rasheed M E H, Youseffi M, Parisi L and Sefat F 2023 Complementary and alternative medicine (CAM) use for cancer patients *AIP Conf. Proc.* **2872** 1

[3] Ring A and Parton M 2016 *Breast Cancer Survivorship: Consequences of Early Breast Cancer and its Treatment* (Cham: Springer)

[4] Sagen A, Kaaresen R, Sandvik L, Thune I and Risberg M 2014 Upper limb physical function and adverse effects after breast cancer surgery: a prospective 2.5-year follow-up study and preoperative measures *Arch. Phys. Med. Rehabil.* **5** 875–81

[5] Akca M, Ata A, Nayır E, Erdogdu S and Arıcan A 2014 Impact of surgery type on quality of life in breast cancer patients *J. Breast Health* **4** 222–8

[6] American Cancer Society 2017 *Chemotherapy for breast cancer* (American Cancer Society) (https://cancer.org/cancer/breast-cancer/treatment/chemotherapy-for-breast-cancer.html). Accessed 2018

[7] American Cancer Society 2018 *Targeted therapy for breast cancer* (American Cancer Society) (https://cancer.org/cancer/breast-cancer/treatment/targeted-therapy-for-breast-cancer.html). Accessed 2018

[8] Loibl S and Gianni L 2017 HER2-positive breast cancer *Lancet* **389** 2415–29

[9] breastcancer.org 2019 *Immunotherapy* (breastcancer.org) (https://breastcancer.org/treatment/immunotherapy). Accessed 2020

[10] breastcancer.org 2019 *Tecentriq* (breastcancer.org) (https://breastcancer.org/treatment/immunotherapy/tecentriq). Accessed 2020

[11] Atakan Z 2012 Cannabis, a complex plant: different compounds and different effects on individuals *Ther. Adv. Psychopharmacol.* **2** 241–54

[12] Kiskova T, Mungenast F, Suvakova M, Jager W and Thalhammer T 2019 Future aspects for cannabinoids in breast cancer therapy *Int. J. Mol. Sci.* **7** 1673

[13] Miller N and Oberbarnscheidt T 2020 The impact of cannabidiol on psychiatric and medical conditions *J. Clin. Med. Res.* **12** 393–403

[14] Blessing E, Steenkamp M, Manzanares J and Marmar C 2015 Cannabidiol as a potential treatment for anxiety disorders *Neurotherapeutics* **12** 825–36

[15] Massi P, Solinas M, Cinquina V and Parolaro D 2013 Cannabidiol as potential anticancer drug *Br. J. Clin. Pharmacol.* **75** 303–12

[16] Sallaberry C and Astern L 2018 The endocannabinoid system, our universal regulator *J. Young Invest.:* **34**

[17] Rady I *et al* 2018 Anticancer properties of Graviola (*Annona muricata*): a comprehensive mechanistic review *Oxid. Med. Cell Longev.* **2018** 1826170

[18] Qazi A, Siddiqui J, Jahan R, Chaudhary S, Walker L, Sayed Z, Jones D, Batra S and Machal M 2018 Emerging therapeutic potential of graviola and its constituents in cancers *Carcinogenesis* **39** 522–33

[19] Moghadamtousi S, Fadaeinasab M, Nikzad S, Mohan G, Ali H and Kadir H 2015 *Annona muricata* (Annonaceae): a review of its traditional uses, isolated acetogenins and biological activities *Int. J. Mol. Sci.* **16** 15625–58

[20] cancerresearchuk.org 2018 *Graviola (soursop)* (cancerresearchuk.org). (https://cancerresearchuk.org/about-cancer/cancer-in-general/treatment/complementary-alternative-therapies/individual-therapies/graviola). Accessed 2019

[21] Chorlton M, Rees E, Phillips C, Claypole T, Berry N and Row P *Investigation of the Antimicrobial Activity of Culinary and Medicinal Herbs and Spices Against Selected Gastrointestinal Pathogens* (Wales: NHS Wales)

[22] Key E 2014 *Thyme & Oregano, Healing and Cooking Herbs* (North Carolina: Lulu.com)

[23] Kubatka P *et al* 2017 Oregano demonstrates distinct tumour-suppressive effects in the breast carcinoma model *Eur. J. Nutr.* **3** 1303–16

[24] Dhaheri Y, Attoub S, Arafat K, AbuQamar S, Viallet J, Saleh A, Agha H, Eid A and Iratni R 2013 Anti-metastatic and anti-tumor growth effects of origanum majorana on highly metastatic human breast cancer cells: inhibition of NFκB signaling and reduction of nitric oxide production *PLoS One.* **8** e68808

[25] Khalid K, Ahmad A, Khalid S, Ahmed A and Irfan M 2014 Mineral composition and health functionality of zamzam water: a review *Int. J. Food Prop.* **17** 661–77

[26] Shomar B 2012 Zamzam water: concentration of trace elements and other characteristics *Chemosphere* **86** 600–5

[27] Mahmoud H *et al* 2020 Zamzam water is pathogen-free, uricosuric, hypolipidemic and exerts tissue-protective effects: relieving BBC concerns *Am. J. Blood Res.* **10** 386–96

[28] Omar U, Doghaither H, Rahimulddin S, Al-Ghafari A, Zahrani S and Aldahlawi A 2017 *In Vitro* cytotoxic and anticancer effects of zamzam water in human lung cancer (A594) cell line *Cancer J.* **15** 1098–104

[29] Abd-Rabou A, Assirey E, Saad R and Ibrahim H 2018 Metallocenes-induced apoptosis in human hepatic cancer HepG2 cells: the prodigy of zamzam water *Int. J. Pharmacol.* **14** 260–70

[30] Siraj A, Begum R, Melosantos R, Albalawy W, Abboud J, Siraj N and Al-Kuraya K 2019 Zamzam water protects cancer cells from chemotherapy-induced apoptosis via mitogen-activated protein kinase-dependent pathway *Biomed. Pharmacother.* **118** 109376

[31] BBC 2011 *No arsenic in genuine holy water', Saudis say* (BBC) (https://bbc.co.uk/news/uk-england-london-13326566). Accessed March 2021

[32] Xiang Y, Guo Z, Zhu P, Chen J and Huang Y 2019 Traditional Chinese medicine as a cancer treatment: Modern perspectives of ancient but advanced science *Cancer Med.* **8** 1958–75

[33] Fu B, Wang N, Tan H, Li S, Cheung F and Feng Y 2018 Multi-component herbal products in the prevention and treatment of chemotherapy-associated toxicity and side effects: a review on experimental and clinical evidences *Front Pharmacol.* **9** 1394

[34] Li S, So T, Tang G, Tan H, Wang N, Ng B, Chan C, Yu E and Feng Y 2020 Chinese herbal medicine for reducing chemotherapy-associated side-effects in breast cancer patients: a systematic review and meta-analysis *Front Oncol.* **10** 599073

[35] Liu W *et al* 2019 Therapeutic effects of ten commonly used chinese herbs and their bioactive compounds on cancers *Evid. Based Complement Alternat. Med.* **2019** 6057837

[36] Jiao L, Bi L, Lu Y, Wang Q, Gong Y, Shi J and Xu L 2018 Cancer chemoprevention and therapy using chinese herbal medicine *Biol. Proceed. Online.* **20** 1

[37] Guo Y *et al* 2018 Paris polyphylla-derived saponins inhibit growth of bladder cancer cells by inducing mutant P53 degradation while up-regulating CDKN1A expression *Curr. Urol.* **11** 131–8

[38] Li F, Jiao P, Yao S, Sang H, Qin S, Zhang W, Zhang Y and Gao L 2012 Paris polyphylla Smith extract induces apoptosis and activates cancer suppressor gene connexin26 expression *Asian Pac. J. Cancer Prev.* **13** 205–9

[39] Zhang D *et al* 2018 Anti-cancer effects of paris polyphylla ethanol extract by inducing cancer cell apoptosis and cycle arrest in prostate cancer cells *Curr. Urol.* **11** 144–50

[40] Lee M, Yuet-Wa J, Kong S, Yu B, Eng-Choon V, Nai-Ching H, Chung-Wai T and Fung K 2005 Effects of polyphyllin D, a steroidal saponin in Paris polyphylla, in growth inhibition of human breast cancer cells and in xenograft *Cancer Biol. Ther.* **4** 1248–54

[41] breastcancer.org 2019 *Blood marker tests* (breastcancer.org). (https://breastcancer.org/symptoms/testing/types/blood_marker) Accessed 2020

Chapter 5

Medical imaging

5.1 Background

Following the understanding of the elements associated with breast cancer in the previous chapters, chapter 5 describes the topic of medical imaging and its associated aspects. Medical imaging is the visualisation of the inside of the human body using different techniques and it is mainly conducted for an effective clinical examination of a specific disease [1]. Researchers have discussed various imaging modalities and processes that have been heavily in use for the diagnostic and treatment purposes and the improvement of public health. In general, medical imaging can reduce unnecessary courses of action and the right use of medical imaging can result in the avoidance of some surgical procedures [2]. Various imaging modalities are used for diagnostic and treatment purposes and among the widely used imaging techniques are X-ray and ultrasound imaging (USI). Imaging for medical purposes is very effective and even if medical and clinical judgements are sufficient for analysing a disease and its severity and determining the correct treatment, the use of diagnostic imaging techniques cannot be overlooked or suppressed. Medical imaging plays an effective role in the timely confirmation, correct assessment and documentation of many complex diseases, including breast cancer. Medical imaging has an important role in dealing with breast cancer screening, diagnosis and treatment monitoring. Past studies have reported significant evidence that mammography has an effective role in the diagnosis of breast cancer, and it is considered as the gold standard [3]. Other imaging techniques used for breast cancer are ultrasound imaging and magnetic resonance imaging (MRI). Medical imaging plays a vital role in the detection of metastatic lesions even before the appearance of symptoms. Timely detection and diagnosis of breast cancer is essential for controlling the rising rate of breast cancer occurrence and the under-lying factors leading to such rise. The effective follow-up of breast cancer survivors is also very important to avoid recurrence of the disease [4]. However, like diagnosis,

doi:10.1088/978-0-7503-5709-8ch5

treatment and follow-up stages of breast cancer are still under investigation by medical researchers in the context of breast cancer and the role of medical imaging techniques. This review is therefore intended to add to the available literature through the presentation of an integrated view of the role of different types of medical imaging techniques in the simultaneous diagnosis, treatment and follow-up of breast cancer.

5.2 Ionising radiation medical imaging techniques

A range of medical imaging techniques has been developed for improving the outcomes of body imaging in the field of healthcare and medicine. Among these medical imaging modalities, there are various medical imaging techniques used for breast cancer screening, diagnosis and treatment monitoring. In the academic literature it has been identified that several current medical imaging techniques used for breast imaging principally employ low energy and low-resolution approaches, the consequences of which are quite harsh leading to harmful effects. Studies have reported that regular use of medical imaging techniques sometimes can result in false-positive outcomes of imaging, further leading towards overtreatment and unnecessary and invasive follow-up testing [5]. The academic literature has also shown that some of the medical imaging techniques are ultimately leading towards the development of non-invasive methods for tumour location and for improving the efficiency and effectiveness of drug development programmes [6]. Despite some of the negative sides of medical imaging techniques, past researchers have identified the contribution they make in the effective evaluation and adjustment of treatment protocols in real-time situations to assist in the effective reorganization of the cancer drug development process [7, 8]. The academic literature given in this chapter tends to offer details of the different medical imaging techniques that use ionising radiation to generate images used for breast cancer overall assessment at different stages of the medical process. The medical imaging techniques discussed in this review include X-ray, Mammography, and Computed Tomography (CT).

5.2.1 X-ray (conventional radiography)

X-ray is the most conventional medical imaging technique and has been used for many years for different functions [9]. Clinicians use X-rays for diagnosis, monitoring and treatment of various medical conditions. X-rays are a type of electromagnetic radiation with very high energy and short wavelengths, and can pass through the human body as well as many other objects [10]. X-rays can produce clear images of the human body from inside. Medical X-rays are used for generating images to show up abnormalities in bones and other structures and certain tissues inside the human body such as breast tissues. The significance of X-rays has been heavily addressed in past studies with respect to the detection of early-stage breast cancers. Many researchers have recognised X-rays as a primary imaging modality that is highly feasible for breast cancer diagnosis [9]. An X-ray machine produces short bursts of X-rays. As X-rays travel through the body, they also travel through a detector on the other side of the body; the detector then forms an image [11]. In the

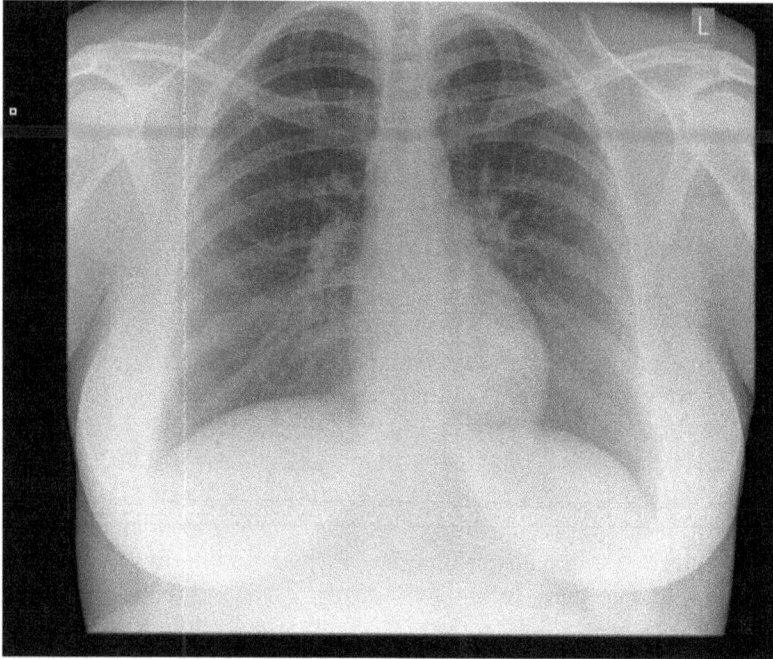

Figure 5.1. Normal chest X-ray of a 23-year-old female in PA view. Reproduced from [15]. CC BY 3.0.

X-rays, images are produced using electromagnetic waves with wavelengths within the range of 0.01 to 10 nanometres (nm) [12]. Electromagnetic waves capture source images of tissues and can convey the information to computer devices attached to an X-ray machine. The technique has a remarkable penetrating ability, which makes it useful for the medical radiography. X-rays have played a significant role in breast cancer screening as an important imaging modality that is highly feasible for breast cancer diagnosis [13]. Chest X-rays are also used to monitor how the disease is responding to treatments and to monitor other conditions, e.g., if there is pneumonia or inflammation in the lungs [14]. Medical X-rays are safe when used with care and, in general, the lowest amount of radiation necessary to get the required results is used. A contrast medium is used in contrast X-rays to show blood vessels and other fluid filled and hollow structures that do not usually show up on X-rays. The following image (figure 5.1) is a normal chest X-ray (CXR) of a young woman in the PA view demonstrating normal shape as well as size of the chest (thoracic) wall and the contents of the thorax [15].

X-rays are categorised into hard and soft X-rays based on the levels of photon energies. High photon energies with short wavelength and great penetrating power are known as hard X-rays. On the other hand, soft X-rays are lower energy with longer wavelength and less penetrating power [16]. Hard X-rays are usually used in medical X-ray imaging. Contrary to past practices, clinicians in the present era have started using X-rays as an integrated part of other medical imaging techniques such as mammography. At the start of the 20th century, X-rays were identified as highly effective medical imaging techniques used for the treatment of breast cancer especially in the surgical removal of breast tumours. However, the technology needed to be refined to provide improved contrasts due to the low density of breast tissues and the weak absorption of standard energy X-rays and the fact that the diagnosis of breast cancer lesions is highly challenging for clinicians, with conventional X-ray methods being only able to capture straight images without any dimensional views. However, modern X-ray images have resolved this concern by presenting two-dimensional as well as three-dimensional views of the various human body parts [17]. An X-ray is a painless and quick test used to examine the bones and teeth, chest and abdomen. Chest X-rays are reported to be the most commonly used medical imaging technique in emergency departments [126]. On X-rays, bones and dense tissue show up as white, muscles and fat show up as shades of grey and air shows up as black. The most common views of a chest X-ray are the posteroanterior (PA) view and lateral view. The anatomy of the chest is well demonstrated in the PA view. The PA view of the chest examines the bony thoracic cavity, the heart and the lungs, the great vessels and the mediastinum. The PA and lateral chest X-ray are a standard chest examination and are usually read together. However, a lateral chest X-ray is more difficult to interpret [18]. A lateral chest X-ray is taken from the side of the patient, and it similarly gives valuable information on the bony thoracic cavity, the heart, the lungs, the pericardium, the pleura, the mediastinum and the upper abdomen.

5.2.2 Mammography (mammogram)

Mammography is recognised as the gold standard imaging method used for breast cancer detection [3]. Mammography is a simple X-ray examination of the human breast, and it refers to the specific type of X-ray imaging which produces images based on a low dose of X-ray system specifically designed for the creation of detailed images of the human breast. Mammography is performed on a specific X-ray machine through which each breast is X-rayed separately. During the mammography examination, the breast is positioned on a parallel plate and compressed firmly but gently with a plastic puddle. Mammography functions by evening out the breast thickness. The technique also helps in reducing X-ray distribution. The image processing protocol of basic mammography is based on 2D views of the breast [19]. In a routine screening mammography, two X-rays are taken at different angles, head to foot (craniocaudal (CC)) view and angled side (mediolateral oblique (MLO)) view [20]. The CC view and MLO view are the standard views on mammograms. The importance of using mammograms is that they can detect breast cancer in women with or without signs and symptoms of the disease. Mammograms can spot cancers that are too small to be seen or felt. However, basic digital mammography is not identified as a useful tool for the determination of benign and malignant tumours with high-level certainty. For this reason, false-negative (when a mammogram looks normal whereas cancer is present) and false-positive (when a mammogram looks abnormal whereas no cancer is present) results may occur using mammography.

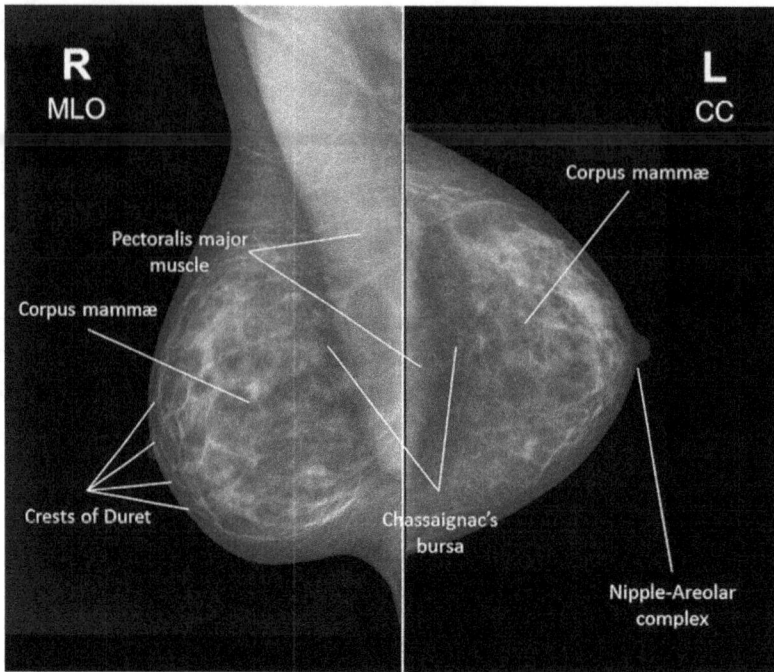

Figure 5.2. Labelled normal mammograms. Reproduced from [21]. CC BY 3.0.

In order to deal with such complicatedness, advanced medical imaging techniques have been developed such as the following three recent advances in mammography:

- Digital mammography or full-field digital mammography (FFDM).
- Computer-assisted diagnosis or computer-aided detection (CAD).
- Breast tomosynthesis or digital breast tomosynthesis (DBT), also known as three-dimensional (3D) mammography.

However, other advanced medical imaging techniques have also been developed and used besides mammography for the overall assessment of breast cancer. Figure 5.2 shows annotated mammograms of a normal breast [21].

5.2.3 Computed tomography (CT)

Computed tomography (CT), which is also known as computerised tomography or computerised axial tomography (CAT), is a medical imaging technique that uses X-rays to obtain medical images. A CT scanner has an X-ray source and a detector as well as a flat motorised bed for patients to lie on. The flat bed passes through a large rotating ring of the scanner. The ring does not surround the whole body, but a small section of the body as the patient passes through it. When the CT scan rotates, the X-ray source and the detector both rotate, and a series of X-ray pictures of the body are taken from different angles. A computer is then used to put the pictures

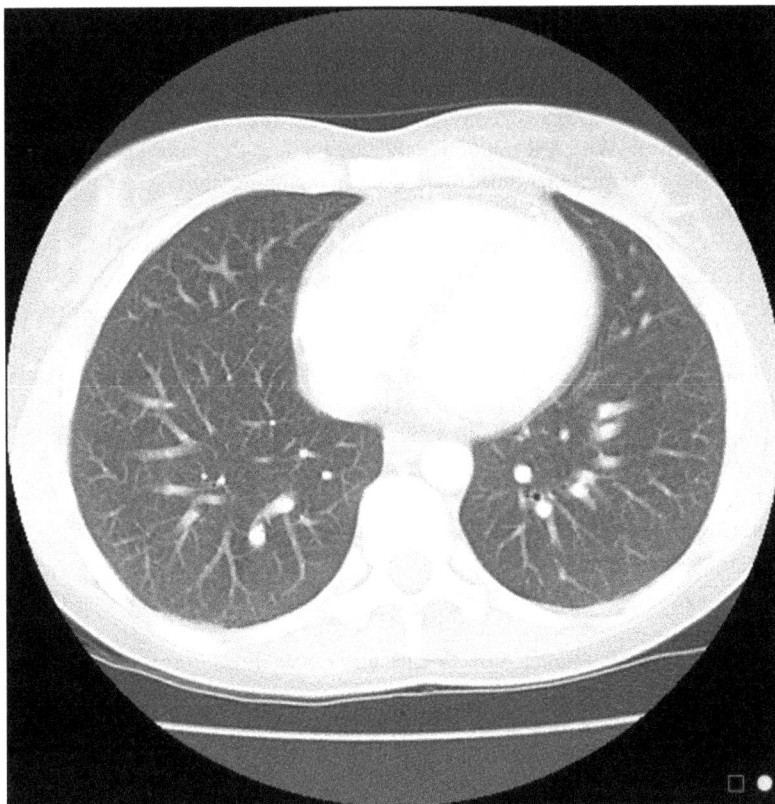

Figure 5.3. Normal chest on CT (lung window) in a 35-year-old female. Reproduced from [24]. CC BY 3.0.

together to produce a detailed 3D image [22]. A contrast medium is a special dye that is given to the patient to improve the image quality. A CT scan plays an important role in breast cancer diagnosis, treatment and monitoring including examination of the tumour size during and after treatment. The contrast medium of the CT scans of the chest can show up the tissues and blood vessels around the breast cancer, which helps one to see if the tumour can be removed by surgery [23]. The following image (figure 5.3) shows a CT image of a normal chest appearance (axial lung window) of a 35-year-old woman [24].

References

[1] Haidekker M 2013 *Medical Imaging Technology* (New York: Springer)
[2] WHO 2017 *Diagnostic imaging* Report WHO_DIL_01.1 (WHO) (http://who.int/diagnosti-c_imaging/en/). Accessed 2018
[3] Andreea G, Pegza R, Lascu L, Bondari S, Stoica Z and Bondari A 2012 The role of imaging techniques in diagnosis of breast cancer *Curr. Health Sci. J.* **37** 55
[4] Bucchi L *et al* 2016 Recommendations for breast imaging follow-up of women with a previous history of breast cancer *Radiol. Med.* **12** 891–6

[5] Kwon S and Lee S 2016 Recent advances in microwave imaging for breast cancer detection *Int. J. Biomed. Imaging* **2016** Article ID 5054912 26

[6] Karam A 2016 Breast cancer posttreatment surveillance: diagnosis and management of recurrent disease *Clin. Obstetr. Gynecol.* **59** 772–8

[7] Houssami N, Given-Wilson R and Ciatto S 2009 Early detection of breast cancer: overview of the evidence on computer-aided detection in mammography screening *J. Med. Imag. Radiat. Oncol.* **53** 171–6

[8] Zi C, Ruocco R, Perrone V, Bruzzese D, Tommasielli G, Laurentiis M D, Cammarota S, Arpino G and Arpino G 2017 Imaging tests in staging and surveillance of non-metastatic breast cancer: changes in routine clinical practice and cost implications *Br. J. Cancer* **116** 821–7

[9] Islam M, Kaabouch N and Hu W 2013 A survey of medical imaging techniques used for breast cancer detection *IEEE Int. Conf. Electro-Inform. Technol.* **EIT 2013** 1–5

[10] Martz H, Logan C, Schneberk D and Shull P 2016 *X-Ray Imaging: Fundamentals, Industrial Techniques and Applications* (Boca Raton, FL: CRC Press)

[11] NHS UK 2018 *X-ray* (NHS UK) (https://nhs.uk/conditions/x-ray/). Accessed 2018

[12] Boundless Physics 2011 *The electromagnetic spectrum* (lumenlearning.com) (https://courses. lumenlearning.com/boundless-physics/chapter/the-electromagnetic-spectrum/). Accessed 2020

[13] Vaughan C 2011 New developments in medical imaging to detect breast cancer *Contin. Med. Educ.* **29** 122–5

[14] breastcancer.org 2016 *Chest x-rays* (breastcancer.org) (https://breastcancer.org/symptoms/ testing/types/xray). Accessed 2018

[15] Bickle I *Normal chest radiograph* (Female radiopaedia.org) (https://radiopaedia.org/cases/ 33225). Accessed 2019

[16] van der Plaats G J 2012 *Medical X-Ray Techniques in Diagnostic Radiology: A Textbook for Radiographers and Radiological Technicians* (Berlin: Springer)

[17] LeVine H 2010 *Medical Imaging* (California: ABC-CLIO)

[18] Gaber K, McGavin C and Wells I 2005 Lateral chest x-ray for physicians *J. Royal Soc. Med.* **98** 310–2

[19] Sree S, Ng E, Acharya R and Faust O 2011 Breast imaging: a survey *World J. Clin. Oncol.* **2** 171–8

[20] CE4RT 2014 *Mammography Review* (Las Vegas: CE4RT)

[21] Pacifici S 2013 *Labeled normal mammograms* (radiopaedia.org) (https://radiopaedia.org/ cases/25751). Accessed 2019

[22] Seeram E 2015 *Computed Tomography: Physical Principles, Clinical Applications, and Quality Control* (Missouri: Elsevier)

[23] cancerresearchuk 2015 *CT scan* (cancerresearchuk). (https://cancerresearchuk.org/about-cancer/cancer-in-general/tests/ct-scan). Accessed 2018

[24] Gaillard F 2010 *Normal chest CT—lung window* (radiopaedia.org). (https://radiopaedia.org/ cases/8095). Accessed 2019

Chapter 6

Non-ionising radiation medical imaging techniques

Chapter 6 discusses non-ionising medical imaging modalities that are used in healthcare including breast cancer patients. The non-ionising medical imaging techniques presented in this chapter are ultrasound imaging (USI) and magnetic resonance imaging (MRI), which are safe and painless available medical modalities used especially for imaging children and other sensitive patient groups.

6.1 Ultrasound imaging (USI)

Ultrasound imaging (USI), which is also known as a sonogram, is identified as one of the most used medical imaging techniques worldwide due to its immense qualities of detection and characterisation of all breast abnormalities. Past studies have highlighted the emerging role of ultrasound imaging for the effective clinical diagnosis of breast cancer. A USI scan generates images of the inside of the human body using high frequency sound waves [1]. The novel developments in ultrasound analysis such as highly sensitive colour Doppler and power Doppler ultrasound machines have further raised the level of ultrasound significance for clinicians as well as patients. Such techniques are capable of detecting the flow inside solid masses through the provision of high-resolution images. USI is widely used in the evaluation of the breast in breast cancer patients, and it is often used after an abnormality is spotted on a screening mammography or when a lump is felt during breast self-examination (BSE) or clinical breast examination. To be noted is that BSE or clinical breast examinations do not provide a definitive diagnosis of breast abnormalities. Likewise, breast ultrasound imaging can generate medical images of the parts of the breast that cannot be seen on a screening mammogram. Importantly, breast ultrasound imaging is also able to find out if a breast lump is a solid mass or a fluid filled cyst [2]. USI involves a small handheld device known as an ultrasound probe which is placed on the breast and moved over. The probe gives off high

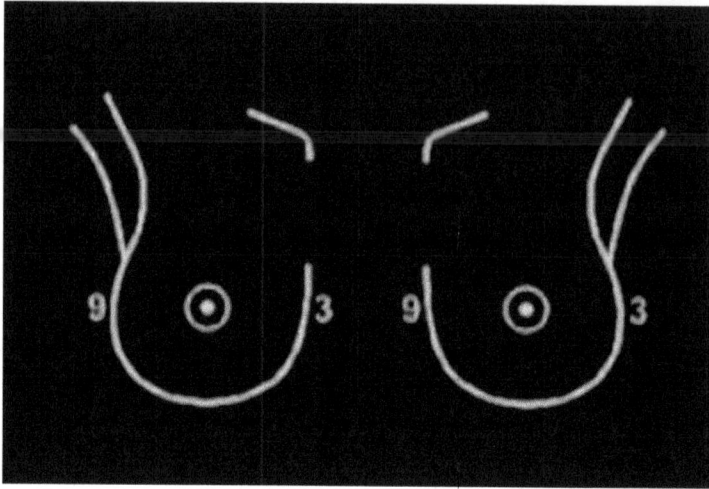

Figure 6.1. Radial and anti-radial scanning with the nipple being in the centre of the clock.

frequency unheard sound waves. The sound waves generate echoes when they bounce off the inside of the breast. The probe then picks up the echoes and turns them into a moving image displayed on a monitor at the same time as the scan is conducted. Ultrasound imaging is also used in breast ultrasound guided biopsy, which is a type of biopsy that uses real-time ultrasound images to visualise abnormalities and lumps in the breast, while a thin needle is inserted into the lump. The tissue removed from the lump is later analysed [3]. The normal scanning technique for breast ultrasound uses the radial and anti-radial scanning planes. Scanning starts at the nipple and radiates out. A clock face or quadrant is used for location description, and for each breast there is a separate clock. The nipple is in the centre of the clock for both breasts as shown in figure 6.1.

Figure 6.2 shows a normal ultrasound image of the right breast of a 50-year-old female with no history of masses or clinical issues [4].

Ultrasound imaging is also reliant on the measurement of the tissue elasticity. The technique is helpful in measuring the elasticity of the breast tissues through an extended form of tissue to provide important diagnostic information that can be used to reduce the number of benign breast biopsies [5]. Automated whole breast ultrasound techniques have been developed for the acquisition of high-quality images in 3D form. This has made ultrasound as unique as the other 3D imaging techniques. The data obtained from the 3D ultrasound screening help in good interpretation at the right time to give the opportunity to reduce the recall rate, sensitivity, specificity and positive predictive value essential when dealing with large volume datasets [6]. Clinicians typically need visual qualitative assessment to analyse the imaging performance and for the comparison of data gathered through different ultrasound imaging probes and modalities, and also to know that the information obtained through ultrasound imaging is gathered using high-level protocol, with the ultrasound technique's protocols being based on complete and open research and

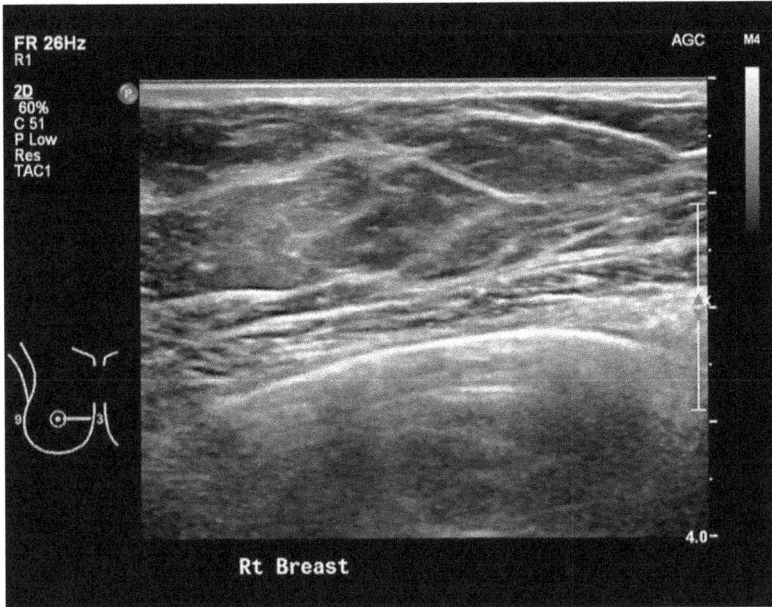

Figure 6.2. Normal breast ultrasound of the right breast at 3:00 o'clock. Reproduced from [4]. CC BY 3.0.

development systems. Researchers have identified that when ultrasound imaging is used with other modalities such as mammography, this can result in the detection of multifocal breast tumours as the capability of ultrasound modality in detecting additional cancers is vital for understanding the overall medical condition [7]. The common USI transducer frequencies are approximately between 2.0 and 15.0 MHz, with 7.5 MHz being typically used for breast ultrasound examination [8]. Likewise, the variety of transducers in different shapes and sizes also help in dealing with the timely diagnosis of a lesion in different types of patients such as pregnant women, men, older patients and others. Ultrasound screening is quite easy to use, and it is a less expensive imaging technique compared to other imaging techniques. The clear imaging of all the breast tissues obtained via ultrasound imaging further makes it a complementary imaging technique with a high level of spatial resolution and real-time imaging useful for the effective detection of breast lesions as well as monitoring of patients [9]. On the contrary, the disadvantages of using the ultrasound imaging technique cannot be undermined while assessing this medical imaging modality. Past studies have shown that ultrasound waves can easily be disrupted by air or gas and for this reason only an ideal imaging technique for air-filled bowel or organs is not possible through the ultrasound technique. Therefore, past studies have identified the challenges associated with the removal of speckle noise in order to retain the significant image characteristics. However, modern ultrasound equipment is helpful in dealing with the issues of image quality and diagnostic values in the real time. The ultrasound technique is recognised as one of the most vital techniques in the academic literature used for the detection of breast lesions. The way ultrasound images are generated needs to be assessed in more detail in relation to other imaging modalities such as magnetic resonance imaging (MRI). In the understanding of MRI images, it is necessary to look at the interaction of the beam with the matter, the modes of operating, beam shape and digital processing. The use of ultrasound imaging in the detection of breast cancer at different stages of screening, however, requires further analysis of its mathematical properties and technical aspects. The properties need to be assessed for the effectiveness of modalities individually as well as collectively.

6.2 Magnetic resonance imaging (MRI)

Medical imaging resonance (MRI) has also been identified as an exceptional medical imaging technique, which is very useful in the timely detection of breast cancer. MRI has been treated as both a conventional and modern approach, which is clinically useful for the provision of volumetric three-dimensional anatomical information as well as physiological information [10]. Magnetic resonance imaging (MRI) uses radio waves and a powerful magnetic field to generate very detailed cross-sectional images of the inside of almost any part of the body. MRI is indicative of the increased vascular density and vascular permeability changes occurring in affected breasts. Past studies have reported up to 100% sensitivity for MRI in detecting invasive cancers [11, 12]. MRI scan is painless and is one of the safest available medical procedures [13]. The MRI scanner has a large tube with strong magnets inside. The MRI machine used for breast screening is known as MRI with dedicated breast coils. During the scan, the patient lies face down on a flat table inside the MRI tube, with the breasts hanging down into an opening in the flat table. MRI is used as a supplemental tool with mammogram or sonogram in breast cancer screening in young women with dense breast tissue, high-risk individuals and those who carry BRCA mutations [14]. MRI is used in patients with breast cancer to help measure tumour size and to find out if there are other tumours in the breast. MRI can sometimes be used to tell if a tumour is malignant (cancer) or benign (not cancer). Other advantages of using MRI for medical imaging include its non-ionising nature, which helps in the easy identification of multiple focal cancers, even in situations where the cancer is associated with the chest wall. MRI has also been used for assessing cancer recurrence in women who have undergone lumpectomy and it can be used by clinicians for making detailed observations of breast implants and ruptures [10]. MRI can show up soft tissues very clearly; however, a Gadolinium (Dotarem) contrast (dye) injection is used for MRI scans to detect the pathology of the lesions and to assess their biological features [15]. Gadolinium is a clear colourless fluid that makes the images clearer to show the tissue details and it is injected intravenously before or during the scan. The MRI scan results can help in diagnosing conditions, treatment plans and assessing the effectiveness of previous treatments [13]. Like every other medical imaging technique, the use of MRI is also associated with some image acquisition. Typical breast imaging protocol in MRI modality can be categorised into four stages. In the first stage, scout images are

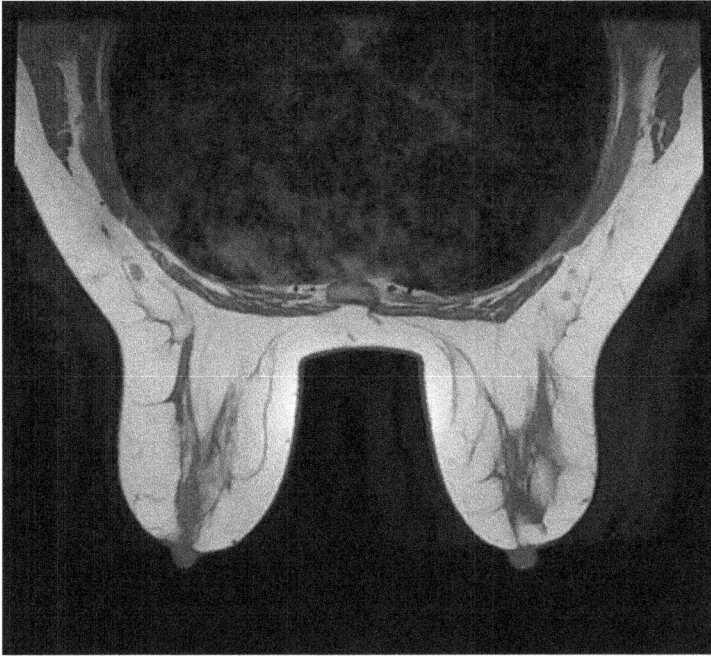

Figure 6.3. Axial T1-weighted MRI image demonstrating left breast intraductal papilloma in a 25-year-old woman with discharge from the left nipple. Reproduced from [18]. CC BY 3.0.

obtained in ($\sim$1 min) and are used for localisation purposes. In the second stage, pre-contrast ($\sim$5–7 min) T1-weighted no-fat suppression and T2-weighted with fat suppression are measured, in addition to a high-resolution 3D T1-weighted fat suppressed gradient-echo sequence. The third stage is of post-contrast, in which 3 to 5 volume acquisitions are obtained in $\sim$10 min. When such images are obtained, the pre-contrast and post-contrast images are compared and must have identical parameters for allowing subtraction. The last stage of image acquisition is analysis of subtraction of pre-contrast and post-contrast images for the identical image parameters with an aim to identify enhanced lesions. The enhancement patterns are used for making the evaluation of dynamic contrast. Analysis is further carried out through maximum intensity projection (MIP). Studies have highlighted that there is a need to have a set of contrast-enhanced pulse sequences at different phases for acquiring identical images [16, 17]. Figure 6.3 shows an axial T1-weighted (T1W) MRI image of a 25-year-old woman with discharge from the left nipple, suggesting intraductal papilloma (small benign tumour that has formed in the left milk duct in the breast).

Researchers have also identified the risks and limitations associated with MRI protocols for provision of effective MRI scanning. Although the MRI process itself is painless it may involve certain aspects, yet it may lead to higher levels of discomfort for patients. These protocols include three key steps focusing on screening procedures, information to subjects upon termination of the session, and the

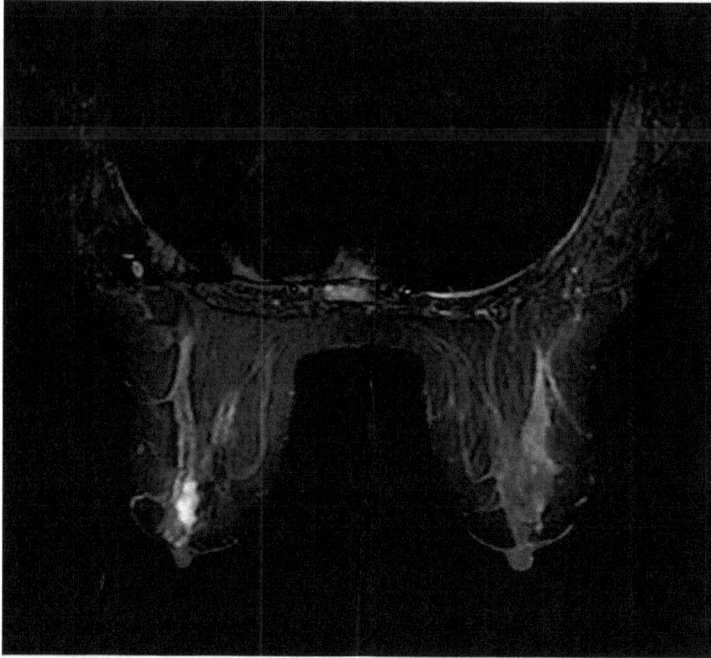

Figure 6.4. Left breast intraductal papilloma MRI (axial T2 FatSat) image of the same patient in figure 6.3. Reproduced from [18]. CC BY 3.0.

provision of disposable earplugs or ear protection against loss of hearing. MRI has been thoroughly investigated for its safety and biological effects due to the exposure of patients to electromagnetic fields under this medical imaging technique. The biological effects and safety in using MRI has been addressed in past studies and it has been mentioned that unnecessary examinations need to be avoided for reducing the risk levels, and the employment of precautionary principles have further been suggested [19, 20]. Figure 6.4 shows an axial T2-weighted (T2W) fat-saturated (FatSat) MRI image of the same patient in figure 6.3 that has left breast intraductal papilloma showing up to 90% to 100% accuracy.

References

[1] Sree S, Ng E, Acharya R and Faust O 2011 Breast imaging: a survey *World J. Clin. Oncol.* **2** 171–8
[2] Shetty M 2015 *Breast Cancer Screening and Diagnosis: A Synopsis* (New York: Springer)
[3] NHS UK 2016 *Diagnosis* (NHS UK). (https://nhs.uk/conditions/breast-cancer/diagnosis/). Accessed 2018
[4] Hacking C 2019 *Normal breast mammography (tomosynthesis) and ultrasound* (radiopaedia. org). (https://radiopaedia.org/cases/65325). Accessed 2019
[5] Barr R 2010 Real-time ultrasound elasticity of the breast: initial clinical results *Ultrasound Q.* **26** 61–6

[6] Drukker K, Sennett C and Giger M 2014 Computerized detection of breast cancer on automated breast ultrasound imaging of women with dense breasts *Med. Phys.* **41** 012901

[7] Brem R, Lenihan M, Lieberman J and Torrente J 2015 Screening breast ultrasound: past, present, and future *Am. J. Roentgenol.* **204** 234–40

[8] Nadrljanski M and Murphy A 2010 *Ultrasound frequencies* (radiopaedia.org) (https://radiopaedia.org/articles/8664). Accessed 2020

[9] Kaur K 2013 Digital image processing in ultrasound images *Int. J. Rec. Innov. Trends Comput. Commun.* **1** 388–93

[10] Andreea G, Pegza R, Lascu L, Bondari S, Stoica Z and Bondari A 2012 The role of imaging techniques in diagnosis of breast cancer *Curr. Health Sci. J.* **37** 55

[11] Orel S and Schnall M 2001 MR imaging of the breast for the detection, diagnosis, and staging of breast cancer *Radiology* **220** 13–30

[12] Mann R, Kuhl C and Moy L 2019 Contrast-enhanced MRI for breast cancer screening *J. Magn. Reson. Imaging* **50** 377–90

[13] NHS UK 2018 *MRI scan* (NHS UK). (https://nhs.uk/conditions/mri-scan/). Accessed 2018

[14] Barh D 2014 *Omics Approaches in Breast Cancer: Towards Next-Generation Diagnosis, Prognosis and Therapy* (New York: Springer)

[15] Wyld L, Markopoulos C, Leidenius M and Senkus-Konefka E 2018 *Breast Cancer Management for Surgeons: A European Multidisciplinary Textbook* (Cham: Springer)

[16] Hendrick R 2008 Breast magnetic resonance imaging acquisition protocols *Breast MRI* (New York: Springer) pp 135–69

[17] Ron P 2011 *Breast MRI: Pulse Sequences, Acquisition Protocols, and Analysis* (Nashville: Vanderbilt University Medical Center)

[18] Rasuli B 2019 *Intraductal papilloma (breast MRI)* (radiopaedia.org). (https://radiopaedia.org/cases/66992). Accessed 2020

[19] Hartwig V, Giovannetti G, Vanello N, Lombardi M, Landini L and Simi S 2009 Biological effects and safety in magnetic resonance imaging: a review *Int. J. Environ. Res. Public Health* **6** 1178–798

[20] Formica D and Silvestri S 2004 Biological effects of exposure to magnetic resonance imaging: an overview *Biomed. Eng. Online* **3** 11

Chapter 7

Radionuclide medical imaging techniques

Chapter 7 discusses the use of nuclear medicine or radionuclide imaging modalities used for patients with breast cancer and other types of cancer as an effective diagnostic imaging modality. The nuclear medicine techniques presented in this chapter include positron emission tomography (PET) and single-photon emission computed tomography (SPECT), in addition to hybrid medical imaging modalities. The chapter also discusses topics of medical image analysis, DICOM standard and Merge PACS, and medical image quality. The chapter ends by presenting the use of artificial intelligence (AI) for the enhancement of breast cancer medical imaging techniques as a new area of research and development. It should be noted that some sections of this chapter about the use of AI for breast cancer imaging were presented at the University of Bradford's 2023 Yorkshire Innovation in Science and Engineering Conference and have been submitted as a conference paper for publication with the Institute of Electrical and Electronics Engineers (IEEE) [1].

7.1 Introduction

Radionuclide imaging or nuclear medicine scanning is a medical imaging technique used to visualise the inside of the body by using a small amount of radioactive chemicals called radiotracers that are injected into the body [2]. The radiotracers accumulate in the body, and they give off energy in the form of gamma rays. Gamma cameras are then used to detect this energy and generate detailed images. Radionuclide imaging is a very effective diagnostic technique as it can show the structure and the physiological function of different parts of the body. Researchers have identified the effectiveness of radionuclide imaging techniques in visualising the lesion sites as well as the reflection of specific biological and functional imaging features of the lesions. The features of these lesions include metabolic activities, the status of receptors, as well as perfusion, etc [3]. Radionuclide-based methods are identified as molecular imaging modalities which have potentials in the detection and characterisation of breast lesions. Such techniques have enhanced the ability of clinical procedures for gene expression, protein expression as well as for investigating cellular biochemistry [4]. Researchers have emphasised the role of nuclear medicine in monitoring the therapy response, the progression of the disease, as well as recurrence of the cancer [5]. Moreover, clinicians have investigated the use of radionuclide imaging techniques with other modalities such as MRI or CT to produce hybrid imaging modalities to increase the resolution and sensitivity of this specific medical imaging technique which is vital to increase diagnostic confidence. The radionuclide imaging techniques used for breast cancer include various forms of nuclear medicine scans such as positron emission mammography (PEM), breast-specific gamma imaging and scintimammography, which is also called nuclear medicine breast imaging or molecular breast imaging (MBI). MBI is not a screening tool for breast cancer but a supplemental investigative tool to investigate a breast abnormality detected on mammography. During the exam, the radioactive tracer (technetium-99m (Tc-99m) sestamibi) is given to the patient intravenously [6]. Imaging must start immediately after the radioactive tracer injection, and it takes about 40 min. A special gamma camera is used to scan the breast from several angles. The radioactive tracer used is taken up more by the cancer cells than the normal breast tissue. MBI can help in reducing unnecessary procedures and it is defined as an appropriate imaging modality in patients with dense breast tissue [2]. Past studies have highlighted that MBI is superior to normal screening mammography in detecting breast tumours by up to 3 times in patients with dense breast tissue [7]. However, MBI is an expensive imaging modality, with the procedure taking longer, in addition to higher radiation doses. Past studies have confirmed the role of nuclear medicine in breast cancer assessment and that radionuclide imaging is efficient in highlighting the risk of complications with cardio functions and the assessment of cardiotoxicity resulting from chemotherapy and chemoradiotherapy in breast cancer patients [8]. Evidence is also present for the effectiveness of this imaging technique for the axillary sentinel lymph node (SLN) detection in breast cancer [9].

7.1.1 Positron emission tomography (PET)

A positron emission tomography scan is a nuclear medicine scanning technique that uses radioactive tracers to show the activity of the tissues and organs inside the body [10]. A PET scan can detect cancer cells and tissues before they show up on other imaging techniques. A PET scan is useful for evaluating breast cancer in patients diagnosed with the disease, it can also determine how far the disease has spread to other parts of the body and how well the disease is responding to treatments. In most PET scans the radioactive tracer used is known as fluorodeoxyglucose (FDG). FDG is glucose with one oxygen atom replaced by a fluorine-18 (^{18}F). Fluorine-18 (^{18}F) is a radioactive isotope of fluorine, and it is an important source of positrons. The chemical activity of the cancer cells is higher than healthy cells because cancer cells grow at a faster rate, therefore cancer cells take up more of the FDG tracer than normal tissue. The FDG tracer settles in the cancer cells and releases positrons that can be detected by the PET scan. During the procedure, the radioactive tracer is given to the patient through an intravenous injection and then the patient lies still on a flatbed that is moved into a large circular scanner. A special camera is then used to scan the body to produce detailed 3D images [11]. In general, a PET scan scans the whole body which can help to see if cancer has spread to other parts of the body. The PET scan used for breast imaging is known as positron emission mammography (PEM). The positron detecting plates are like the compression system used in mammography; however, the PEM scan does not require compression. During the scan, the breast is placed gently, and two small movable flat detectors are used by PEM cameras. The flat detectors are pressed against the breast directly [10]. PEM has demonstrated a better sensitivity, particularly for small lesions' detection [12]. Hybrid imaging has been introduced to combine PET with CT or with MRI into one single machine. When radionuclide imaging is combined with CT or MRI, special views are produced due to image fusion [11]. The image fusion shows information from two different scans on one image allowing more accurate information. The following image (figure 7.1) is an axial PET/CT fusion image of a 35-year-old lactating woman with lymphoma (swollen lymph nodes and lumps). The image shows normal physiological Fluorine-18 (^{18}F) FDG uptake in both lactating breasts [13].

To be noted is that the process of producing breast milk (lactation) for pregnant or women giving birth, is normal. Hormones signal the mammary glands to produce milk. For staging workup of lymphoma, Fluorine-18 (^{18}F) FDG PET-CT was performed in this patient. Hybrid imaging machines can provide more precise diagnoses than the two imaging techniques carried out separately. PET scans measure the function of the body tissues and organs to help in evaluating how well they are

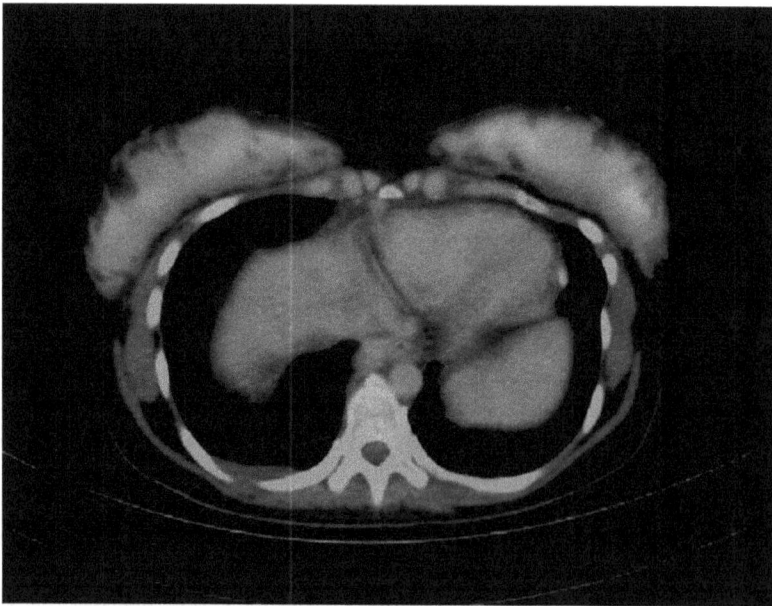

Figure 7.1. Axial Fluorine-18 (^{18}F) FDG PET/CT fusion image. Reproduced from [13]. CC BY 3.0.

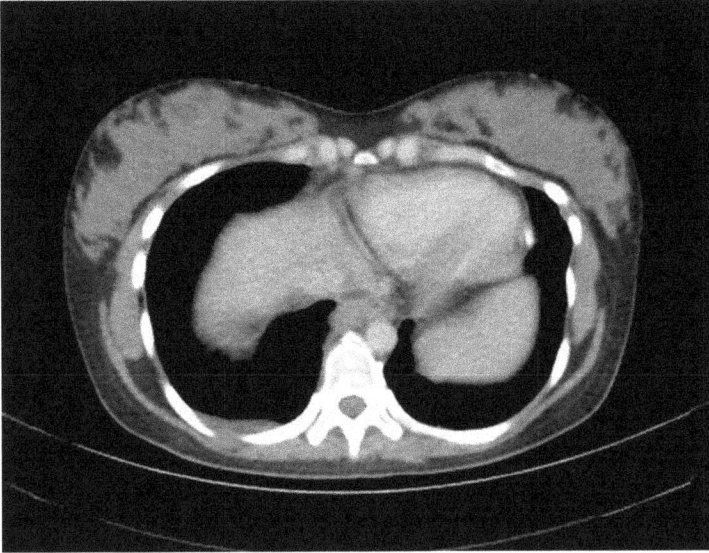

Figure 7.2. Axial contrast-enhanced CT in the portal venous phase. Reproduced from [13]. CC BY 3.0.

functioning. The following image (figure 7.2) is the axial contrast-enhanced CT in the portal venous phase of the same patient (figure 7.1) [13]. It should be noted that in the portal venous phase the contrast agent is mostly in the veins.

While CT scans provide excellent anatomical information, a PET/CT scan can reveal information about both the function and the structure of the body tissues and organs during one single scanning session. The registered images can be viewed through a focused colour display for any cross-sectional view [14]. In breast cancer imaging PET/CT scans are carried out to detect the disease and are used as part of staging to check for metastasis of the cancer to other areas of the body. PET/CT is also used to assess the treatment effectiveness besides breast cancer recurrence after treatment. Likewise, PET/MRI hybrid imaging combines metabolic information of the body tissues and organs provided by PET scanning and excellent soft tissue contrast provided by MRI. The excellent soft tissue contrast provided by MRI is very important as PET imaging on its own provides little anatomical information with low spatial resolution, which makes it difficult to localise the lesion and give the correct evaluation of the spread of the disease to the surrounding tissues. PET/MRI can also provide an improved differentiation of malignant and benign breast tumours [15].

7.1.2 Single-photon emission computed tomography (SPECT)

Single-photon emission computed tomography (SPECT) is a radionuclide imaging technique that uses a radioactive tracer to generate pictures of the body's internal structures and organs. The radioactive tracer is given to the patient intravenously, usually 20 min or more before the scan [16]. The body tissues that are more active will take up the radioactive substance more than the normal tissues. The SPECT scanner is a large circular machine. During the scan, the patient lies on a table inside the machine. A special camera that rotates around the body is used to produce 3D images. These images can show colours of the body parts that have absorbed less of the radioactive substance and the body parts that have absorbed more. A SPECT scan provides functional information of the selective absorption of the injected radioactive tracer by the cancer cells. This information helps one to find tumours that are missed by other imaging techniques. However, with the images produced by SPECT it is hard to measure the precise location of the tracer uptake as these images do not provide enough anatomical framework. Therefore, a SPECT scanner has been combined with a CT scanner in one single scanning device to produce hybrid SPECT/CT scanners, as a CT scan can offer precise anatomical information [17]. SPECT/CT as a combined image can provide information in more detail; it allows more accurate identification of lesions by combining the functional information provided by radionuclide imaging SPECT and the anatomical information provided by CT. In patients with breast cancer, SPECT/CT is used for the diagnosis, staging and follow-up of the disease, due to the increased diagnostic specificity and sensitivity of the radionuclide imaging SPECT and the anatomical information provided by CT [18].

7.2 Medical image analysis

The role of medical image analysis has been significantly identified by medical researchers to identify the effectiveness of these technologies in helping clinicians for the effective risk assessment of cancer, detecting tumours, diagnosis and treatments of different types of cancer. Researchers have highlighted that medical image analysis is able to conduct quantitative image analysis of breast cancer. Their ability to analyse breast images has been explained through a range of characteristics such as morphological attributes, textural attributes and kinetic attributes. Breast image analysis techniques help in segmenting, future extracting, classified designing, biomechanical modelling, registering images along with the attribute of correcting motions [19]. Examination of the effectiveness of medical image analysis techniques has further substantiated the ability of these techniques and assisted clinicians with effective medical image registration and fusion processes. Medical image analysis techniques are also used for the diagnosis and the subsequent follow-up stages in order to optimise the decision-making process about appropriate therapies needed for dealing with patients' conditions. These techniques have been identified as helpful for making the fusion of different imaging modalities by combining the main characteristics of each of modality. However, clinical researchers have confirmed the need to carry out trial-based studies in order to confirm the effectiveness of medical image analysis techniques for dealing with breast cancer patients experiencing different stages [20].

7.3 DICOM standard and Merge PACS

Digital Imaging and Communications in Medicine (DICOM) is the international standard protocol used for managing and transmitting medical images and related information exchanged between medical imaging modalities from various healthcare centres and computers to be used in healthcare, research and education. With DICOM, high resolution digital images generated by DICOM-compliant modalities (such as CT, MRI and USI) are integrated into a Picture Archiving and Communication System (PACS) imaging system (such as Merge PACS). Merge PACS is used for processing, reading, reporting and displaying medical images and it is used in this work for presenting the medical images of the discussed cancer cases obtained from various hospitals [21, 22].

7.4 Medical image quality

Table 7.1 shows the spatial resolution of the medical images obtained via the medical imaging modalities discussed in this work.

Spatial resolution refers to the pixel numbers used for the construction of the digital images. The quality of the digital images is determined by the spatial resolution with the ability to distinguish between two adjacent objects. Spatial resolution in digital imaging depends on the size of the pixels used. Large pixels are unable to distinguish between two adjacent objects in comparison to smaller size pixels. Digital images composed of more pixels are higher spatial resolution images of the same dimension and imaging part [23].

7.5 Artificial intelligence (AI) and breast cancer imaging

Medical imaging modalities such as mammography can help detect breast cancer especially in women who do not have any signs and symptoms of the disease. However, past studies have highlighted that false-negative and false-positive results may occur using basic digital mammography [24]. In order to solve such breast imaging issues, advanced medical imaging techniques were developed such as full-field digital mammography (FFDM), computer-aided detection (CAD) and digital breast tomosynthesis (DBT) for better visualisation of the breast tissue; although these advanced techniques still had false results [25, 26]. Additionally, while medical images are read by radiologists or those reporting images, it is possible that they may misread medical images and fail to diagnose medical conditions or cancers which may have serious consequences for patients. Various factors such as a radiologist's lack of knowledge and other human errors (including errors of overreading) may contribute to missed diagnoses [27]. The following images (figure 7.3) are the unilateral

Table 7.1. Spatial resolution.

Medical imaging modality	Spatial resolution
X-ray	High
Computed tomography (CT)	Very high
Mammography	High
Ultrasound imaging (USI)	Very high
Magnetic resonance imaging (MRI)	High
Radionuclide imaging (PET, SPECT)	Low

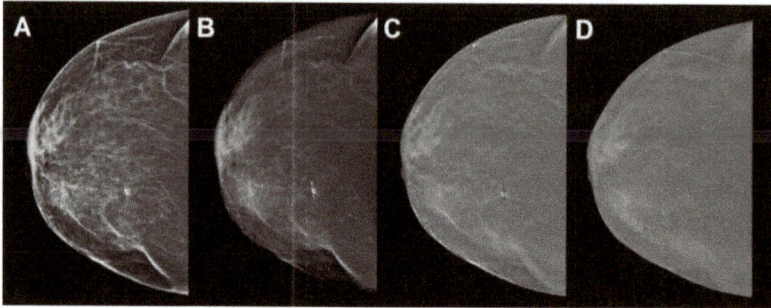

Figure 7.3. Unilateral mammograms of a middle-aged woman with invasive breast cancer in the right breast. (A) Right 2D mammogram craniocaudal (CC) view. (B), (C) and (D) RCC breast tomosynthesis images (different slices).

mammograms of a middle-aged woman with invasive breast cancer in the right breast demonstrating digital breast tomosynthesis being added to standard mammography.

The use of AI in medical diagnostics, particularly in medical imaging such as breast cancer imaging, can significantly improve a patient's quality of care and help minimise misdiagnoses and achieve high accuracy [28, 29]. A standard mammogram is performed in combination with tomosynthesis to produce 3D images and it was approved to be optionally used in the National Health Service (NHS) breast screening programme (BSP) in the UK. NHS mammographers require certain training before using digital breast tomosynthesis in the clinic. Radiologists and those reporting images are also required to take training before they start reporting digital breast tomosynthesis images. DBT as well as FFDM and CAD allow improved breast visualisation; however, these techniques still suffer from a high number of false-positive results per analysed image. Moreover, medical images taken via these advanced techniques may also miss tumours that are present in patients due to human error and cancers may not be visible to radiologists as a result of many factors including tiredness or loss of concentration [27]. In the last few years, scientific studies have concentrated on the application of AI in the field of breast cancer imaging. AI in breast cancer imaging by the use of machine learning algorithms to detect changes in breast mammograms with fewer missed tumours has been developed to help radiologists in breast cancer screening programmes through various ways including replacing at least one of the mammography readers. AI can offer many advantages due to the fact that it is a computer image recognition, and it does not get tired or lose concentration. AI use within the NHS BSP is currently under discussion by the UK National Screening Committee (UK NSC). Researchers in the UK have already secured funding from the government through the AI in Health and Care Award in partnership with the National Institute for Health Research (NIHR) and NHSX to test and evaluate the use of AI for breast cancer screening in NHS hospitals [30]. Past studies have reported that the use of AI in the detection of breast cancer showed improved diagnostic performance in comparison with radiologists as human readers, as well as substantial improvements in the performance of the readers when assisted by AI [28, 29]. According to the UK NSC review on the use of AI for image

Case 1:

Case 2:

Case 3:

Case 4:

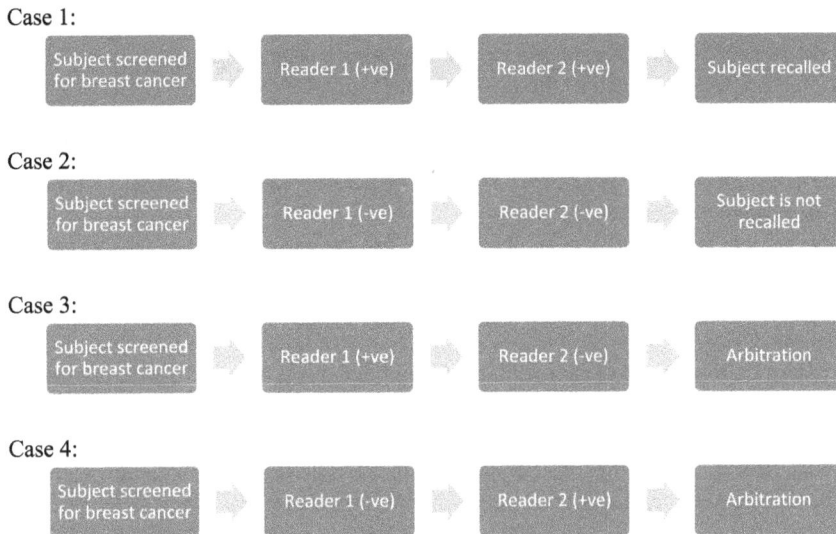

Figure 7.4. The current breast screening pathway in the UK. Case 1 when the subject tests positive by both readers, she is recalled for further tests. Case 2 when the subject tests negative by both readers, she is not recalled for further tests. Case 3 and 4 when the subject tests positive by either reader 1 or reader 2, arbitration is employed.

analysis in breast cancer screening, the current breast screening pathway in the UK is explained as in the following image (figure 7.4) [31].

According to the UK NSC it is explained that AI is proposed to be used in the current breast screening pathway as the following:

- To be used as a pre-screening tool removing clear normal cases.
- To completely replace reader 1 and reader 2.
- To replace reader 2.
- To aid decision-making for one or both readers.

Likewise, more research is needed to provide evidence and approve each proposed AI use in the current breast screening pathway. It should be noted that researchers in the UK have secured funding from the government to do more research on the application of AI in breast cancer screening within the NHS. However, this work proposes that the application of AI strongly needs to be used as an assistive tool in medical imaging, not to totally replace human readers and radiologists with focus on gradual transformation considering all risk areas that may be caused by AI.

References

[1] Rasheed M E H, Youseffi M, Zaernia A and Parisi L 2023 *Artificial Intelligence and Medical Imaging for Breast Cancer Screening* (Piscataway, NJ: IEEE)

[2] Prakash D 2014 *Nuclear Medicine: A Guide for Healthcare Professionals and Patients* (New York: Springer)

[3] Silov S, Taşdemir A, Ozdal A, Erdoğan Z, Başbuğ E, Arslan A and Turhal O 2014 Radionuclide imaging for breast cancer diagnosis and management: is technetium-99m tetrofosmin uptake related to the grade of malignancy? *Hell. J. Nucl. Med.* **17** 87–9

[4] Specht J and Mankoff D 2012 Advances in molecular imaging for breast cancer detection and characterization *Breast Cancer Res.* **14** 206

[5] Greene L and Wilkinson D 2015 The role of general nuclear medicine in breast cancer *J. Med. Radiat. Sci.* **62** 54–65

[6] Lille S and Marshall W 2018 *Mammographic Imaging* (Philadelphia, PA: Lippincott Williams & Wilkins (LWW))

[7] Vaughan C 2011 New developments in medical imaging to detect breast cancer *Contin. Med. Educ.* **29** 122–5

[8] Lapinska G, Kozlowicz-Gudzinska I and Sackiewicz-Slaby A 2012 Equilibrium radionuclide ventriculography in the assessment of cardiotoxicity of chemotherapy and chemoradiotherapy in patients with breast cancer *Nucl. Med. Rev. Cent. East. Eur.* **15** 26–30

[9] Mudun A *et al* 2008 Comparison of different injection sites of radionuclide for sentinel lymph node detection in breast cancer: single institution experience *Clin. Nucl. Med.* **33** 262–7

[10] Pluchinotta A 2015 *The Outpatient Breast Clinic: Aiming at Best Practice* (New York: Springer)

[11] NHS UK 2018 *PET scan* (NHS UK) (https://nhs.uk/conditions/pet-scan/). Accessed 2018

[12] Veronesi U, Goldhirsch A, Veronesi P, Gentilini O and Leonardi M 2017 *Breast Cancer: Innovations in Research and Management* (Cham: Springer)

[13] Qureshi P 2019 *Normal physiological FDG uptake in lactating breasts* (radiopaedia.org). (https://radiopaedia.org/cases/69438). Accessed 2019

[14] Dhawan A 2011 *Medical Image Analysis* (Hoboken, NJ: Wiley)

[15] Umutlu L and Herrmann K 2018 *PET/MR Imaging: Current and Emerging Applications* (New York: Springer)

[16] mayoclinic.org *SPECT scan* (mayoclinic.org). (https://mayoclinic.org/tests-procedures/spect-scan/about/pac-20384925). Accessed 2018

[17] Kim C and Zukotynski K 2017 *SPECT and SPECT/CT: A Clinical Guide* (Stuttgart: Thieme)

[18] Sergieva S, Mihaylova I, Alexandrova E, Fakirova A and Saint-Georges A 2015 Clinical application of SPECT-CT in breast cancer *Arch. Cancer Res.* **4** 3

[19] Giger M, Karssemeijer N and Schnabel J 2013 Breast image analysis for risk assessment, detection, diagnosis, and treatment of cancer *Annu. Rev. Biomed. Eng.* **2013** 327–57

[20] El-Gamal F, Elmogy M and Atwan A 2016 Current trends in medical image registration and fusion *Egypt. Inform. J.* **17** 99–124

[21] dicomstandard.org 2021 *DICOM* (dicomstandard.org) (https://dicomstandard.org) Accessed 2021

[22] Bidgood W, Horii S, Prior F and Syckle D 1997 Understanding and using DICOM, the data interchange standard for biomedical imaging *J. Am. Med. Inform. Assoc.* **4** 199–212

[23] Athanasiou L, Fotiadis D and Michalis L 2017 Propagation of segmentation and imaging system errors *Atherosclerotic Plaque Characterization Methods Based on Coronary Imaging* (Cambridge, MA: Elsevier) 151–66

[24] Roman M, Hofvind S, Euler-Chelpin M and Castells X 2019 Long-term risk of screen-detected and interval breast cancer after false-positive results at mammography screening: joint analysis of three national cohorts *Br. J. Cancer* **120** 269–75

[25] Kim S, Moon W, Seong M, Cho N and Chang J 2009 Computer-aided detection in digital mammography: false-positive marks and their reproducibility in negative mammograms *Acta Radiol.* **50** 999–1004

[26] Mahoney M and Meganathan K 2011 False positive marks on unsuspicious screening mammography with computer-aided detection *J. Digit. Imaging* **24** 772–7

[27] Bruno M, Walker E and Abujudeh H 2015 Understanding and confronting our mistakes: the epidemiology of error in radiology and strategies for error reduction *RadioGraphics* **35** 1668–76

[28] Gao Y, Geras K, Lewing A and Moy L 2019 New Frontiers: an update on computer-aided diagnosis for breast imaging in the age of artificial intelligence *AJR. Am. J. Roentgenol.* **212** 300–7

[29] McKinney S *et al* 2020 International evaluation of an AI system for breast cancer screening *Nature* **577** 89–94

[30] NHS UK 2021 *AI in health and care award winners* (NHS UK) (https://nhsx.nhs.uk/ai-lab/ai-lab-programmes/ai-health-and-care-award/ai-health-and-care-award-winners/). Accessed 2022

[31] Freeman K, Geppert J, Stinton C, Todkill D, Johnson S, Clarke A and Taylor-Phillips S 2022 *Use of Artificial Intelligence for Mammographic Image Analysis in Breast Cancer Screening* (UK National Screening Committee)

IOP Publishing

Breast Cancer and Medical Imaging

Mohammed Erkhawan Hameed Rasheed and Mansour Youseffi

Chapter 8

Breast cancer and medical imaging clinical case studies

Chapter 8 discusses clinical case studies and medical images taken via different medical imaging techniques used in cancer detection and diagnosis in addition to appropriate genetic testing to identify specific gene mutations that cause breast cancer. This chapter also presents an introduction to genetic counselling as well as clinical case studies information governance. It should be noted that some sections from this chapter about the dense breast tissue case were presented at the *2021 IEEE 17th International Colloquium on Signal Processing & Its Applications (CSPA)* and have been submitted as a conference paper for publication with the Institute of Electrical and Electronics Engineers (IEEE) [1].

8.1 Information governance

When working on studying and publishing clinical case studies, the names of the patients, dates of birth and hospital numbers as well as any direct or indirect identifiers of all the clinical cases are all deleted. Each case investigated with the analysis of medical images taken via various medical imaging modalities are completely anonymised. Only the minimum amount of data required for research purposes are recorded such as the age of the patient, gender, ethnicity, etc, and all are managed with the guidance outlined in the information governance requirements [2] with explicit consent given in writing and verbally stated clearly and unmistakably from all of the participants for genetic testing, living cancer patients themselves, family members in the cases of deceased cancer patients, and consent on behalf of children at least from one parent in the cases of children, to confirm that the law and best practice is complied with in regard to handling information.

doi:10.1088/978-0-7503-5709-8ch8

8.2 Introduction to genetic counselling

Genetic testing or genomic testing is mainly carried out to diagnose patients with rare and genetic (hereditary) health conditions and some cancers such as breast cancer. In the case of breast cancer, the test is carried out to find out the chances of a female developing the disease, and also to find out whether she carries a specific gene mutation that could be inherited by her children [3]. Genetic counselling sessions are run by genetic counsellors, and at the appointment the patient's family history of breast cancer and other types of cancer are discussed in detail. The appointment begins by drawing out the patient's family history as a pedigree. The information provided by the patient is used to draw a pedigree to assess the patient's family history so that the patient is able to better understand the diagnoses of different types of cancer that have been reported in the patient's both maternal and paternal sides. The role of genetic counselling is explained to the patient by the counsellor and they assess the probability that cancers may have been caused in the patient's family by inheriting a gene change linked to an increased risk of certain cancers. It is explained to the patient that there is a possibility that the family history of cancer is caused by some specific gene changes or mutations in cases where the patient has a known family history and all the types of cancer seen in the family are known, or if the patient belongs to a specific community that is known of having cancer occurring more frequently among them than in the general population. In cases where the patient has an uncertain family history that does have several members diagnosed with cancers, a full genetic testing is offered. In general, if there are two close relatives of a patient's same family side who have had the same type of cancer or related types of cancer, and they were diagnosed before the age of 50, then this is considered as a strong family history [4]. It is explained to the patient that inherited breast cancer and other related types of cancer are mainly linked to mutations in the genes, BRCA1 and BRCA2. It is also explained that a genetic test is usually available to determine if the patient has BRCA1 and BRCA2 mutations and to find out if the patient is at a higher risk of getting the disease. At the appointment, the counsellor also talks to the patient about the results of genetic testing. It is explained to the patient that women who receive a positive BRCA result have an increased risk of developing breast cancer. It is also explained that there is an increased risk of developing ovarian cancer during one's lifetime. The management options available are also discussed with the patient in case the patient has a positive result, which can be either extra breast surveillance or risk reducing surgery. If they discover that the patient carries a BRCA gene change they would recommend yearly MRI scans from age 30 until 49, and mammograms from age 40. The other management option would be a double mastectomy to remove any remaining breast tissue, which is a major surgery and often a difficult decision for women to make. In general, these options would be discussed with the patient later and the patient is referred to the appropriate teams to discuss further. A positive result would mean that the patient's children would be at 50% risk and from the age of 18 they can request genetic testing. It would also mean that the patient's siblings could also get a test. It is also explained to the patient that when this genetic test is carried out, there is a possibility of receiving a genetic test result called a variant of uncertain significance, a VUS. This would mean that the laboratory found a change in a BRCA gene, but it is uncertain if this alteration is the cause for the patient's diagnosis of cancer. With this finding, they would reassess the patient's cancer risk based on this result and recommend the appropriate screening based on the patient's family history. It is explained to the patient that sometimes these variants are reclassified in time as more is known about them. It is usually suggested that if the patient does receive a VUS result then it is worth ringing the genetics department in a few years' time to see if it has been reclassified. At the end of the appointment if the patient is happy to go ahead with the types of above-mentioned testing, then the patient has to sign the consent form so as the hospital can go ahead with the required procedures.

8.3 Dense breast tissue case

A 30-year-old female patient with dense breast tissue and previous breast mass and a strong family history of breast cancer and other types of cancer was referred to see a genetic counsellor for possible genetic testing. A blood sample was taken from the patient to find out if there are any hereditary gene mutations that might have caused cancer to run in her family. A full BRCA gene test was therefore carried out to see if she has any of the known breast cancer risk genes. The results revealed that the patient is not affected and that she does not have any significant changes in the BRCA1 and BRCA2 genes. Receiving a negative BRCA1 and BRCA2 result is reassuring, since these are the two high risk breast and ovarian cancer genes that are known. This has decreased this family member's risk of developing breast cancer, and the revised assessment now places her breast cancer risk to that of other normal women. This result also means that her daughters and any future children will not be at risk of inheriting a BRCA gene change from her. Although there was no detection of any known pathogenic changes in the BRCA1 or BRCA2 genes of this patient, it does not exclude the possibility of the cancer cases found in her family being BRCA1 and BRCA2 related.

8.3.1 Medical history of the patient

The past medical history of the patient included details of treatment of a benign tumour (fibroadenoma), which was surgically removed from the patient's left breast when she was 15 years old. The reason behind receiving surgical removal of the breast lesion was the patient's strong family history of breast cancer and other types of cancer. Malignant transformation of fibroadenomas is usually rare; however, women with fibroadenomas and a strong family history of breast cancer are investigated with a high suspicion for malignancy, especially in middle-aged women [5]. In general, fibroadenomas are formed with the overgrowth of the breast's glandular tissue and fibrous tissue, and are usually found in women aged 15 to 35. Fibroadenomas are very common with an incidence rate of about 18% to 20% [6]. The hormone levels of women can affect fibroadenomas and can become larger in size during gestation or smaller after the menopause. Some women have one fibroadenoma while others have multiple fibroadenomas in the same breast or in both breasts. Fibroadenomas are usually painless and often found on physical exams. Ultrasound imaging is the best medical imaging modality for looking for fibroadenomas as they may not show up on mammography. Ultrasound imaging is also effective in mammographically dense breast tissue [7]. Following the genetic test results, the patient was referred to have mammography and ultrasound imaging.

8.3.2 Breast imaging reporting and data system (BI-RADS)

Breast imaging reporting includes information about breast density, the presence or absence of breast masses, in addition to lesion size and location. Breast Imaging-Reporting and Data System (BI-RADS) is the quality assurance and risk assessment tool established by the American College of Radiology (ACR) [8]. The tool provides a breast imaging lexicon for mammography, ultrasound and MRI. According to the BI-RADS atlas, the mammography breast composition categories are four categories; (A) mostly fatty breast tissue, (B) scattered fibroglandular breast tissue, (C) heterogeneously dense breast tissue and (D) extremely dense breast tissue. On the other hand, BI-RADS assessment categories are seven (0 through to 6); BI-RADS 0 means incomplete and additional imaging testing is needed; BI-RADS 1 means negative, i.e., no masses; BI-RADS 2 means noncancerous (benign) finding; BI-RADS 3 means benign with low probability of malignancy; BI-RADS 4 means suspicious for malignancy; BI-RADS 5 means highly suggestive of malignancy; and BI-RADS 6 means malignancy [9].

8.3.3 Mammography of the patient

The patient was referred for a mammogram to monitor and detect any breast lesions that the patient might have and in case cancer does develop at an early stage due to the fact that the patient has a strong family history of breast cancer and other types of cancer. Women from families that have breast cancer, ovarian cancer, in addition to some other types of cancer found among them in one or more than one generation are typically considered to be at a higher risk of getting breast cancer. Figures 8.1 and 8.2 show the mammograms of the patient. The mammography standard views are bilateral craniocaudal (CC) and mediolateral oblique (MLO) views. Figure 8.1 shows the mammography of the patient in the right craniocaudal (RCC) view and the left craniocaudal (LCC) view showing extremely dense breast tissue.

In the craniocaudal (CC) view the image shows the entire part of the breast. The nipple is clearly depicted in this view. The fat tissue appears as a dark strip because fat is radiolucent, i.e., it permits the passage of X-rays. The mammography of the patient demonstrated extremely dense breast tissue (BI-RADS category D) which reduced the sensitivity of the mammogram. No obvious speculated masses, suspicious grouped microcalcifications, architectural distortion or nipple retraction could be seen bilaterally. Figure 8.2 shows the mammography of the patient in the right mediolateral oblique (RMLO) view and left mediolateral oblique (LMLO) view. The image in the mediolateral oblique (LMLO) view shows most of the breast tissue in the upper outer quadrant and the axilla.

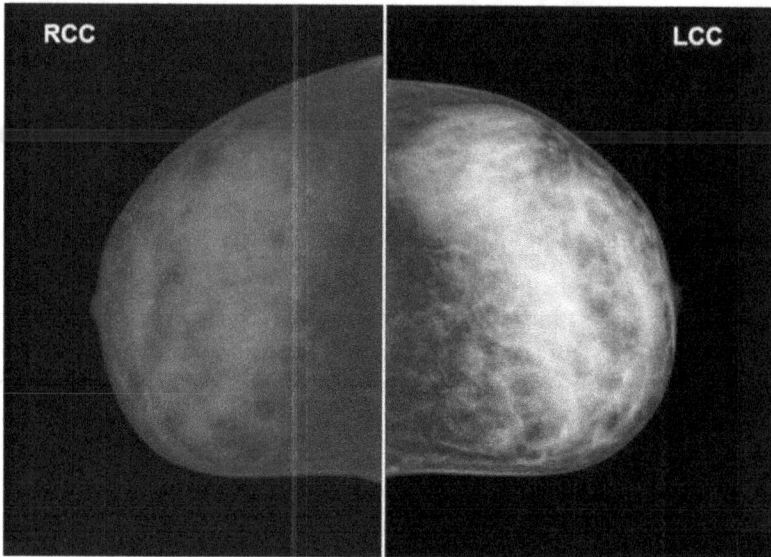

Figure 8.1. Breast screening mammography in craniocaudal (CC) views of the patient demonstrating extremely dense breast tissue.

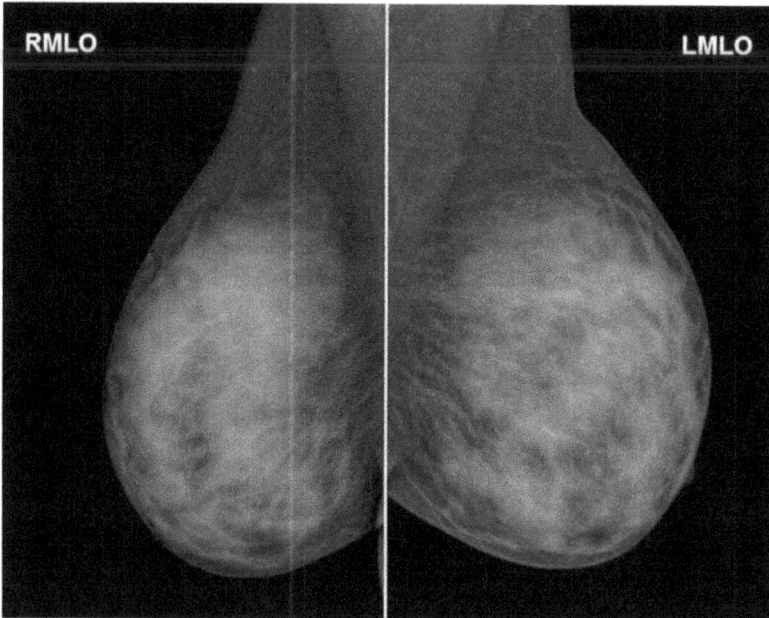

Figure 8.2. Mammograms of the patient in mediolateral oblique views showing extremely dense breasts.

The axilla demonstrated no enlarged lymph nodes. The mammography showed no evidence of any microcalcification or breast masses or any obvious abnormality. The patient's breast imaging reporting and data system (BI-RADS) assessment was therefore category 0 (BI-RADS 0), which means imaging is incomplete, not clear and more tests are needed. Ultrasound imaging was therefore recommended due to dense breast tissue.

8.3.4 Ultrasound imaging of the patient

The patient was scanned at the same site and multiple selected ultrasound images of her breasts were compared to her mammography results dated one day earlier. The ultrasound imaging results showed heterogeneous background echotexture of both breasts. The results also demonstrated a bi-lobed hypoechoic (solid) with inhomogeneous echotexture but with well-defined margin and no associated calcification of the right breast lesion as shown in figure 8.3 and measures 1.8 × 0.8 cm seen at 2 o'clock. The right breast lesion was not seen on the breast mammography due to dense breast tissue and it represents a fibroadenoma (a benign breast tumour) given its inhomogeneity with the presence of a hypoechoic component to it. The normal right nipple and the axilla demonstrated no enlarged lymph nodes. On the other hand, ultrasound imaging of the left breast demonstrated a normal left nipple, normal subcutaneous tissue and no left breast masses. Therefore, the patient's breast imaging reporting and data system assessment was BI-RADS 1 for the left breast. BI-RADS 1 means the test result is normal.

8.3.5 Treatment of the patient

The patient was recommended to have the breast mass removed by surgery based on imaging tests and due to the patient's strong family history of breast cancer and

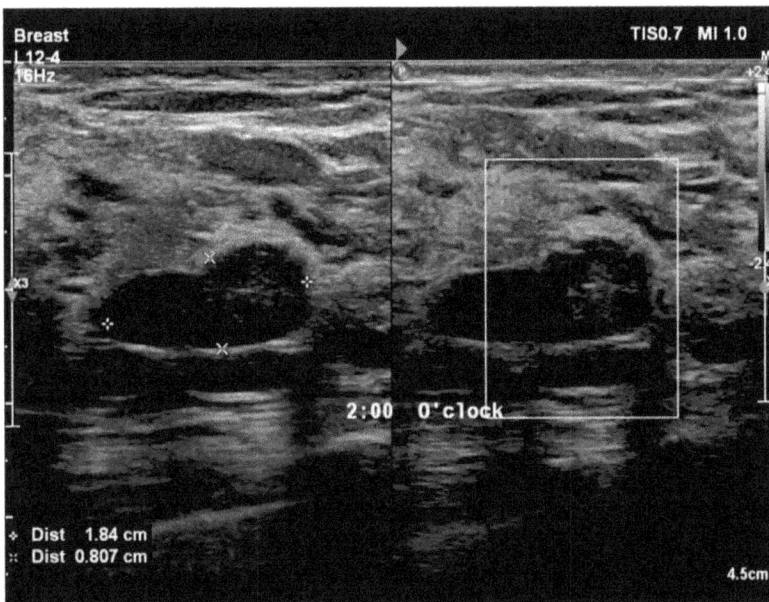

Figure 8.3. Ultrasound imaging of the patient demonstrating a right breast lesion with no architectural distortion surrounding the lesion.

other types of cancer, in addition to the patient's medical history of previous fibroadenoma in the opposite breast at around age 15 which was then removed through surgery. In general, patients with simple fibroadenomas along with no family history of breast cancer are at lower risk of developing breast cancer. If a fibroadenoma is not removed, it is usually followed up with ultrasound imaging every 6 months for 2 years to monitor any increase in size.

8.3.6 Discussion

According to the American College of Radiology (ACR), breast density has an impact on mammographic screening and ACR's instructions are to include their breast density categories information in patients' medical reports [8]. Dense breasts are not related to the size of the breasts, and cannot be self-examined; however, on a mammogram a way to measure the breast density is by measuring the thickness of the breast tissue. ACR's Breast Imaging Reporting and Database System (BI-RADS) includes information on breast density, and it categorises breasts as: (A) mostly fatty, (B) scattered fibroglandular density, (C) heterogeneously dense, and (D) extremely dense. The density of breast can be inherited, i.e., if mothers have dense breast tissue, then daughters are more likely to have dense breasts [10]. In this case study full genetic testing of BRCA1 and BRCA2 was carried out for a female patient with a strong family history of breast cancer and other types of cancer. However, the genetic testing results confirmed that the patient did not have any significant changes in the BRCA1 and BRCA2 genes. Mammography was recommended for the patient, which demonstrated dense breast tissue, BI-RADS category D, i.e., extremely dense, and therefore no pathology could be found. Breast ultrasound was, therefore, recommended following mammography, and the diagnosis obtained using ultrasound imaging indicated a breast mass (fibroadenoma) in the right breast. Due to the patient's strong family history of cancer, and also the patient's previous case of breast fibroadenoma in the left breast at age 15, surgical removal of the breast lesion was recommended based on the imaging tests only, i.e., no biopsy or other imaging tests were carried out. The common sizes of fibroadenomas are 1–3 cm, but they may increase up to 10 cm, and giant fibroadenoma (GFA) are larger than 5 cm [11]. In this case study, the ultrasound imaging technique was identified as an effective medical imaging technique used in the assessment of a patient with dense breast tissue in addition to meeting all the physical and health and safety considerations related to imaging process and procedure.

8.4 Metastatic breast cancer case

The breast cancer case discussed in this section, along with the medical images taken via breast screening mammography in addition to positron emission tomography combined with a computed tomography (PET/CT) scan, are for a middle-aged woman with metastatic breast cancer. Metastatic breast cancer is an invasive breast cancer that has spread from where it started in the breast to other parts of the body. Advanced breast cancers typically spread to the bones (bone metastasis), which was the case with this patient, and to other body parts and organs such as the liver, the lungs and the brain. The patient had breast screening mammography which showed abnormality in her breasts. The patient was subsequently referred for FDG PET/CT evaluation to confirm primary breast cancer and to find out if cancer has spread to other parts of the body. The PET/CT images confirmed primary breast cancer in the right breast and also revealed the occurrence of bone metastasis.

8.4.1 Breast screening mammography

Figure 8.4 shows the breast screening mammography of the patient in the standard bilateral craniocaudal (CC) views showing abnormality in the breasts.

Figure 8.5 shows the breast screening mammography of the patient in the standard right mediolateral oblique (RMLO) view and the left mediolateral oblique (LMLO) view of the patient showing abnormality in the breasts.

8.4.2 Breast cancer and bone metastasis on a PET/CT scan of the patient

The patient subsequently had a PET/CT scan. PET scans use the radioactive tracer Fluorine-18 (^{18}F) FDG which settles in the cancer cells and releases positrons that can be detected by the PET scan. When PET is combined with CT, it can provide information about both the function and the structure of the body tissues and organs. PET/CT is effective for confirming primary breast cancer and staging locally advanced and inflammatory breast cancers. Figure 8.6 shows the axial PET/CT scan of the patient. The image shows the physiological Fluorine-18 (^{18}F) FDG uptake in the right breast and it demonstrates primary breast cancer in the right breast (the arow). Cancer cells have a higher metabolic rate than normal cells, and they show up as bright spots on a PET/CT scan, therefore a PET/CT scan can help in differentiating between

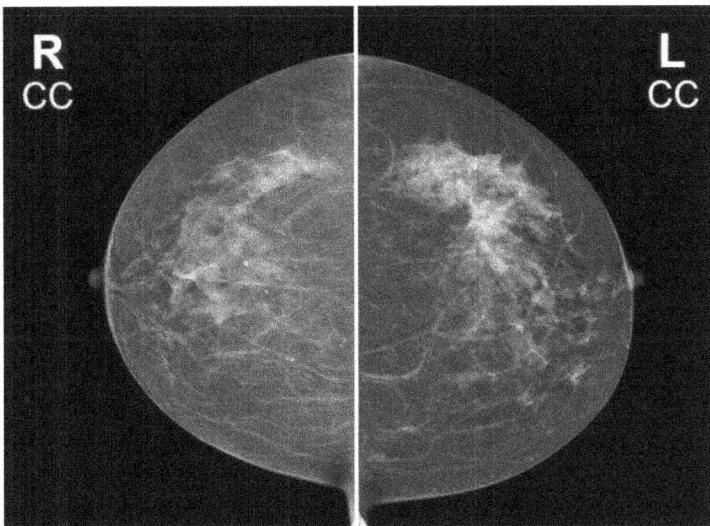

Figure 8.4. Breast screening mammography of the patient in the right craniocaudal (RCC) view and the left craniocaudal (LCC) view with abnormality detected in the breasts.

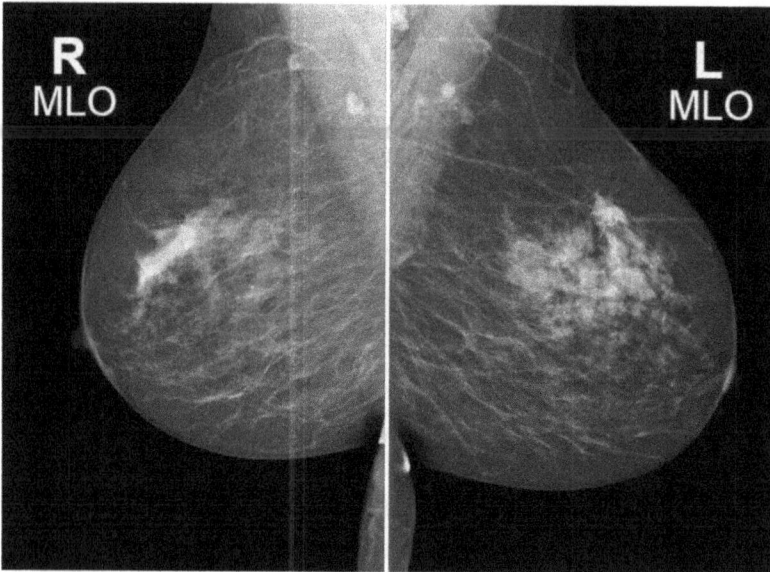

Figure 8.5. Mammograms of the patient in the right mediolateral oblique (RMLO) and the left mediolateral oblique (LMLO) views, demonstrating abnormality in the breasts.

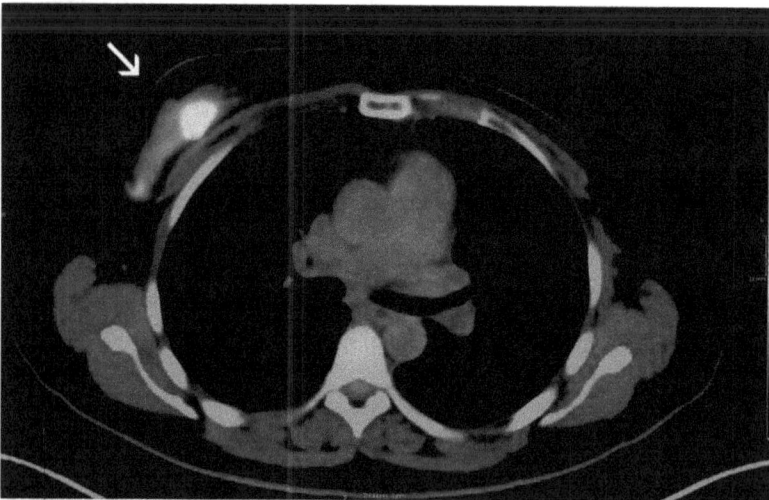

Figure 8.6. Axial PET/CT image demonstrating primary breast cancer in the right breast (the arrow).

cancerous and noncancerous masses. The advantages of a PET/CT scan is that it examines extra-axillary nodes as well as the chest, the abdomen and the bones in one scanning session. A PET/CT scan measures both the anatomy and the metabolic function of the body of the patient and can confirm the primary breast cancer detected on screening mammography. PET/CT is effective to find out if cancer has spread to other parts of the body, and to see if treatment is working.

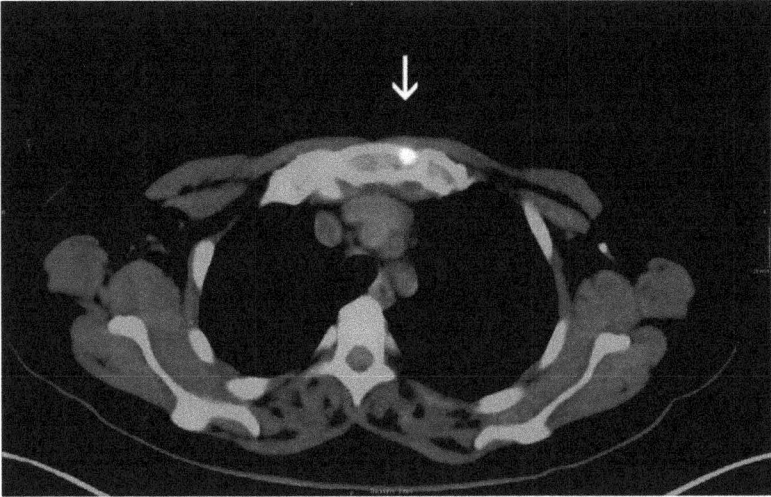

Figure 8.7. Axial PET/CT image demonstrating bone metastasis in the same patient (the arrow).

Figure 8.7 shows the axial Fluorine-18 (^{18}F) FDG PET/CT image, showing bone metastasis in the same patient (the arrow).

8.4.3 Discussion

PET and PET/CT imaging can examine both the cellular metabolism as well as the anatomy of patients with breast cancer fully in one scan and they have shown to be effective in the management of breast cancer in all stages in patients with primary breast cancer and in patients with suspected tumour recurrence. These imaging techniques have shown the capability of detecting early treatment response and help one to choose the most effective treatments. With the PET/CT imaging technique, it is not the architecture of the lesion that is looked at, which is the case with mammography, but rather the metabolic activity of the lesion. A PET scan uses radioactive tracers to show the activity of the tissues and organs in the body and has the ability to detect cancers before they appear on other imaging techniques. PET/CT imaging modality has become a popular imaging technique for the overall assessment of breast cancer. However, the PET/CT system is mostly used in research, and it is not part of routine breast management.

8.5 High grade (G3) triple-negative metaplastic breast cancer

Metaplastic breast cancer (MpBC) is an extremely rare and aggressive subtype of breast cancer that has a poorer clinical outcome in comparison to other breast malignancies. MpBC is typically a triple-negative breast cancer (TNBC); however, MpBC is known to have a worse prognosis and lower survival when compared to the common forms of TNBC. MpBCs are usually high grade and larger in size when they are initially diagnosed, and it is still not understood what exactly causes MpBC. Surgery is typically used for MpBC treatment, along with radiation therapy and chemotherapy. However, MpBCs are more likely to come back after treatment and spread outside the breast to other parts of the body. In this case study, the case of a 50-year-old woman with high grade triple-negative metaplastic breast cancer is presented. This case is a very rare high grade metaplastic breast carcinoma case and it is the only cancer case found among five generations of the patient's family investigated in this work. This case study also includes analysis of a number of medical images of the patient obtained through ultrasound imaging, computed tomography (CT) scan and mammography, in addition to the treatments that the patient has had including surgery and chemotherapy.

8.5.1 Introduction

Metaplastic breast cancer (MpBC) is very rare, comprising 1% or less of all the cases of breast cancer [12]. However, MpBC is an extremely aggressive subtype of breast cancer, and it is known to be difficult to treat. MpBCs are typically triple-negative breast cancers, which means that they are oestrogen-receptor-negative (ER-negative), progesterone-receptor-negative (PR-negative) and HER2-negative. However, when MpBC is compared to the common TNBC types, MpBCs tend to have a poorer prognosis and less disease-free survival [13, 14]. What exactly causes MpBC is still not understood, and MpBCs are typically present as high grade tumours, at a higher tumour stage, and the original tumour is often found larger in size than in other types of breast cancer when they are initially diagnosed due to their rapid growth [15]. 'Grade' is how abnormal the cancer cells look under the microscope and 'stage' is how big the primary cancer is and whether it has spread to other body parts and organs. MpBC is often spread to other parts of the body via the bloodstream and therefore MpBC is less often found in the lymph nodes [16]. The lungs, in addition to the bone and the brain, are the most common sites of distant metastasis of MpBC [17]. An appropriate combination of surgery, radiation therapy and chemotherapy may be used for MpBC treatment. However, some MpBC patients who are initially eligible for surgery may become ineligible due to the progression of the illness before treatment. MpBC patients, especially those with triple-negative, have had a worse response rate to chemotherapy and radiotherapy, and the illness is more likely to come back after treatment and spread outside the breast to other parts of the body [15, 18]. However, MpBC patients without triple-negative may have survival benefit from chemotherapy and radiation therapy [19].

8.5.2 Medical history of the patient

This section discusses the case of a 50-year-old woman with high grade (G3) triple-negative metaplastic breast cancer, including medical history, medical imaging, treatments and the outcomes of the treatments. The medical history of the patient was studied in detail to investigate the causes of her MpBC. The information regarding the patient's medical conditions prior to her MpBC diagnosis included the history of 9 years of acute rheumatic fever. The symptoms of the patient's rheumatic fever included fevers, weakness and painful joints especially her elbow joints, wrist joints, the knees and ankles. At times, the patient had to be carried and turned over due to being unable to even move or stand. The patient had lengthy hospital stays each time, and received treatments to control inflammation as well as the symptoms, including antibiotics and painkillers. It should be noted that the patient was on long-term Penicillin injections. Monthly Penicillin injections are advised in rheumatic fever [20, 21]; however, it has been reported that using Penicillin and antibiotics may increase the risk of cancer [22, 23] and that using antibiotics is linked to increased risk of breast cancer [24]. It is important to mention that studies have also indicated links between rheumatic diseases and cancer and that there is a risk of getting cancer among patients with rheumatic diseases [25, 26].

8.5.3 The patient's family history of cancer

Familial risks of cancer are measured by looking at the medical history of the patient's family members and relatives and investigate if there are cancer occurrences among them. Families usually share similar environments and lifestyle behaviours, in addition to the fact that families have similar genetic backgrounds. The majority of cancer cases (up to 90%) are caused by acquired gene mutations that are caused by environmental factors and lifestyle behaviours (non-inherited). About 3–10% of all cancers are caused by inherited gene mutations which are passed down in families from generation to generation [27]. Cancers caused by non-inherited gene mutations may also appear to run in families when a common environment is shared by them or similar lifestyles. Women from families that have a history of breast cancer and other related types of cancer are at a higher risk of getting the illness. Predictive genetic testing is used to identify if an individual has inherited one of the known cancer risk genes. There are more than 100 cancer risk genes that have been identified linked with an increased risk of breast cancer and other types of cancer [28]. Mutations in BRCA1 and BRCA2 genes are associated with the common inherited breast cancer cases. Typically, it is considered a strong family history if there are two family members who are close relatives of the same family side of a patient and that they were diagnosed with the disease before they reach the age of 50 years. Additionally, and based on findings of the investigations carried out in this study to investigate five generations of the patient's family to find out if other cancer cases are found in her family, it was found that no family members of the patient ever had cancer, and that the patient is the only member of her family that has ever been affected with breast cancer. These results are vital to understand that the patient is not from a family that has a history of cancer and therefore it is less likely that her breast cancer case was caused by inherited gene mutations or gene mutations caused by environmental factors or lifestyles. Therefore, it is suggested that the causes of her rare type of breast cancer are linked to the rheumatic fever and the penicillin treatment that the patient had.

8.5.4 Diagnostic tests

The patient was first admitted to hospital because of pain and swelling in the right breast, where she had a physical breast examination, and an abnormality was noticed in the upper inner quadrant of the right breast. The patient was then referred to the radiology department for breast imaging. The patient had ultrasound imaging, and a 0.9 cm breast mass was found at 2 o'clock in the upper inner quadrant of the right breast as shown in figure 8.8.

Following ultrasound imaging, the patient was referred for a computed tomography (CT) scan to obtain detailed images. CT scans are often used to clarify the location of a tumour and to find out if cancer has spread to other parts of the body. Figure 8.9 shows a CT scan of the chest (axial lung window) of the patient showing a mass in the right breast (see the arrow).

Figure 8.10 shows a CT scan of the chest of the patient in coronal (A), sagittal (B) and axial (C) views with IV contrast (C+) demonstrating a mass in the right breast.

Following the medical imaging tests, the patient was referred for a breast biopsy to take a small sample of the breast mass and examine it under a microscope. The mass was biopsied under the guidance of ultrasound imaging. A small metallic clip was placed inside the breast in order to mark the biopsy site. Figure 8.11 shows the mammography of the affected right breast of the patient showing a small metallic clip (see the arrows). Breast metal clips (titanium clips) are not harmful to the body and typically they are removed at the time of breast surgery. However, it is important to discuss implanting titanium markers with patients beforehand, as titanium can cause allergic reactions and complications [29, 30]. The patient received her biopsy results, and the final diagnosis was breast cancer metaplastic carcinoma grade 3 (G3) triple-negative. G3 means that the cancer cells look very abnormal when compared to normal cells and grow more aggressively (high grade cancer).

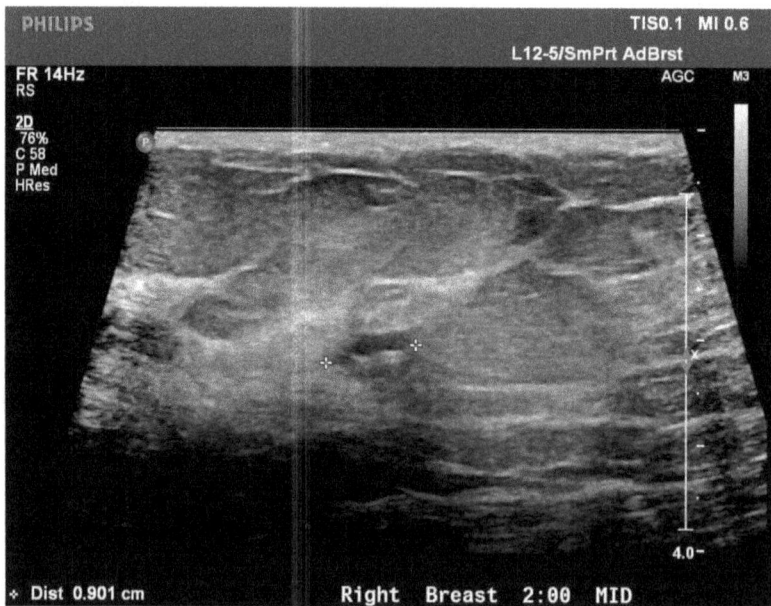

Figure 8.8. Ultrasound image of the patient showing a 0.9 cm hypoechoic mass seen at 2:00 in the right breast.

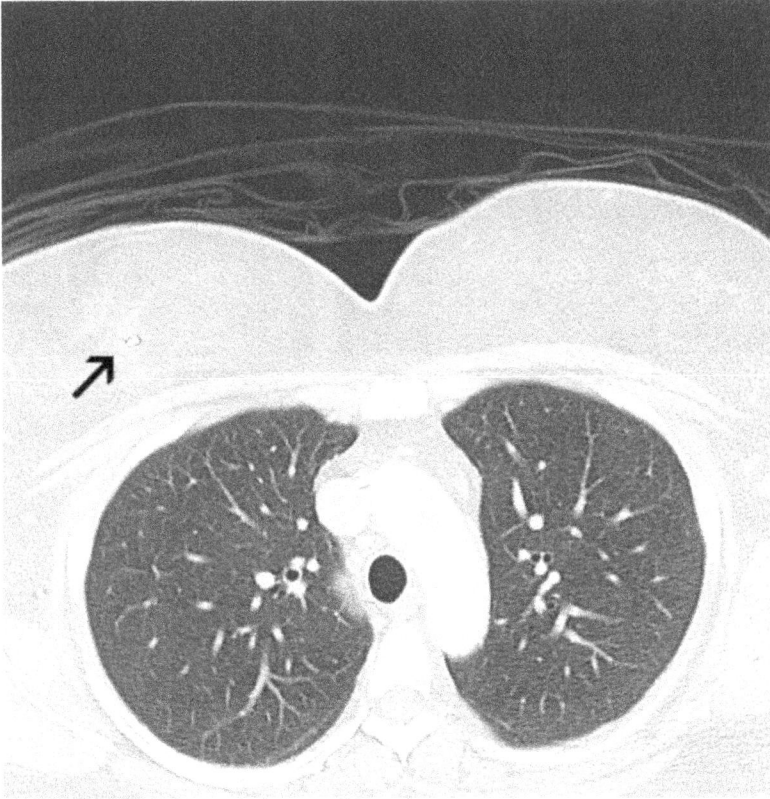

Figure 8.9. CT image (axial lung window) of the chest of the patient demonstrating a mass in the right breast (arrow).

8.5.5 Treatment

The treatments that the patient has had up to the date of authoring this book include surgery and chemotherapy. Following the diagnosis, the patient started to receive neoadjuvant chemotherapy (NAC) regimen for her MpBC, Dose-dense Doxorubicin (Adriamycin)—Dose-dense Cyclophosphamide (Cytoxan) (DDAC) for 4 cycles in addition to DD Paclitaxel (Taxol). Dose-dense (DD) means treatment is given every 2 weeks. One cycle is a 2-week period. Taxol is an effective chemotherapy, and it is commonly used for breast cancer and other types of cancer including ovarian cancer. Taxol is a mitotic inhibitor, and it works by targeting the cancer cells which grow rapidly by mitosis (cell division) and stops them from dividing [31]. Following the NAC, the patient had breast conserving surgery (BCS) in addition to sentinel lymph node biopsy (SLNB). The tumour was surgically removed along with a clear margin or normal tissue around the tumour. SLNB was also carried out as a day case procedure to identify if the first lymph node or nodes contain cancer cells. Figure 8.12 shows the specimen mammograms of the affected

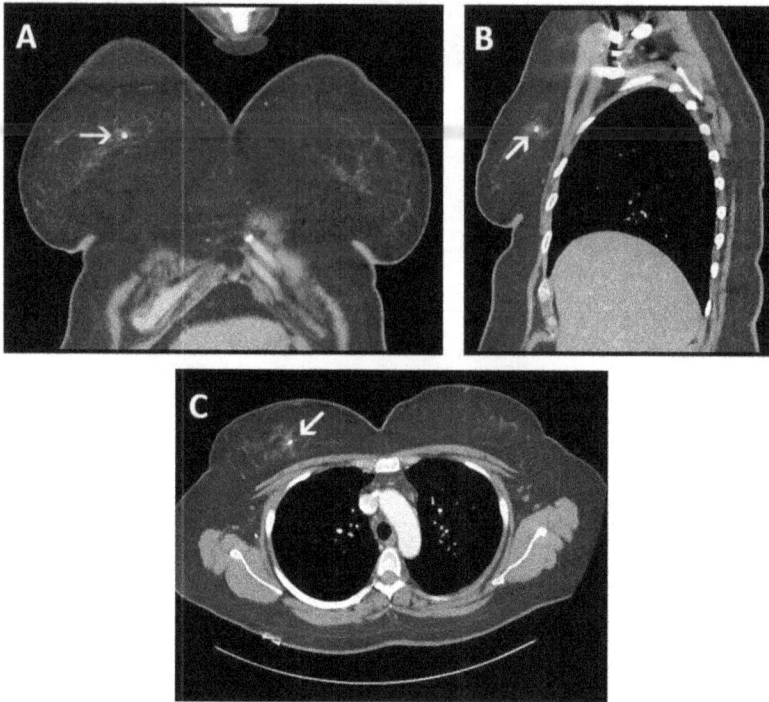

Figure 8.10. Coronal (A), sagittal (B) and axial (C) views of the chest CT with IV contrast (C+) of the patient, identifying a mass in the right breast (see the arrows).

right breast of the patient. Mammography was used for intraoperative margin detection for breast conserving surgery.

Following the surgery, pathology information from the breast tissue that was removed during the surgery was used for staging the patient's breast cancer after her neoadjuvant chemotherapy. The tumour node metastasis (TNM) classification in the patient's pathology report was recorded as ypT1a pN(sn)0. The y prefix is used for staging following NAC. The patient's y-pathological stage ypT1a means the tumour size is more than 0.1 cm but not larger than 0.5 cm. The pathological staging for the patient's regional lymph nodes pN(sn)0 means no cancer cells are found in any nearby nodes. (sn) is confirmed by sentinel node biopsy [32]. The patient was put on adjuvant chemotherapy (adj) to start on adj Capecitabine for 6 months. It is important to mention that breast cancer patients with residual focus of metaplastic carcinoma on pathological testing following NAC are at a higher risk of cancer relapse. Capecitabine is a chemotherapy drug used for breast cancer and other types of cancer. Capecitabine (Xeloda) is a type of chemotherapy that belongs to a class of chemotherapy known as anti-metabolites. Capecitabine is taken as a tablet (orally) and once in the body it is converted to fluorouracil (5-FU), which stops the body cells from DNA synthesis causing the cancer cells to be unable to divide leading to imbalanced cell growth and eventually cell death.

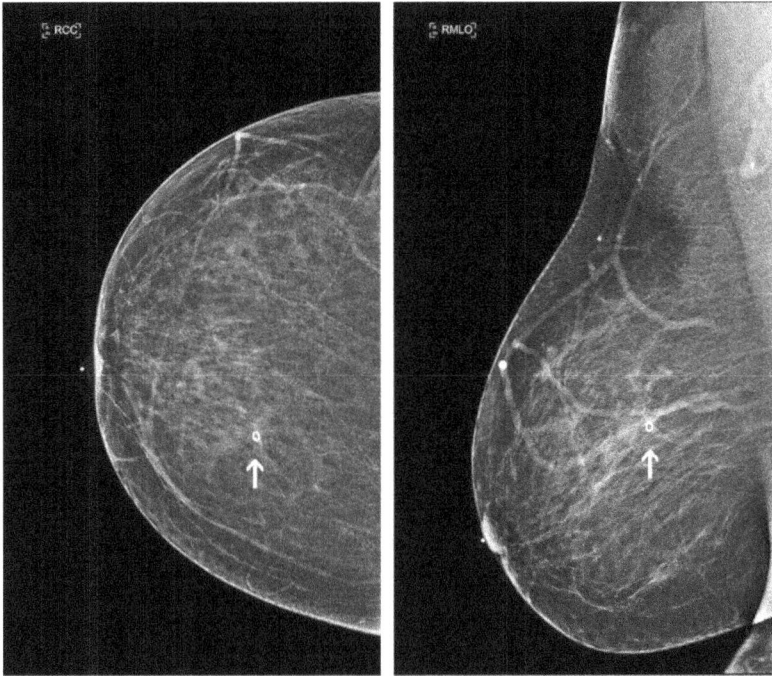

Figure 8.11. Mammograms in the right craniocaudal (RCC) and the right mediolateral oblique (RMLO) views of the patient showing a small metallic clip (see the arrows).

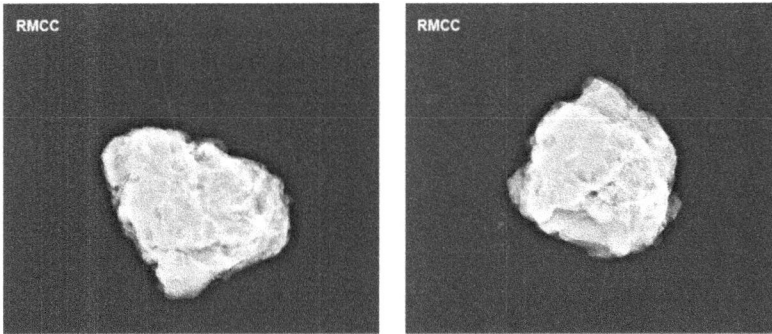

Figure 8.12. Specimen mammograms in the right craniocaudal (RCC) views of the right breast of the patient. The mass was visualised using mammography for intraoperative margin detection for BCS.

8.5.6 Discussion

This work discussed the high grade triple-negative metaplastic breast cancer (MpBC) case of a 50-year-old woman. MpBC is a very rare but very aggressive subtype of breast cancer, and it has a very poor clinical outcome. It is still not known what causes MpBC; however, this patient had a 9-year history of rheumatic fever for which she was put on long-term Penicillin injections prior to her MpBC. The symptoms of MpBC are similar to the common symptoms of breast cancer including changes to the skin of the breast, swelling, pain, etc; however, MpBC may not cause any symptoms. It is therefore very important to report any abnormality when noticed, as the early diagnosis of the disease can have more treatment options with better chances of a cure. The patient in this case study had pain and swelling, and imaging tests demonstrated a mass in the inner upper quadrant of her right breast. The biopsy of the patient was carried out under the guidance of ultrasound imaging and the final diagnosis was metaplastic carcinoma G3 TNBC. Past studies have shown that MpBC typically present high grade and larger in size at the initial time of diagnosis. The patient had NAC prior to her BCS and following her BCS the patient has been put on adjuvant chemotherapy. The pathology report of the breast tissue removed during her BCS showed a tumour size of more than 0.1 cm but not larger than 0.5 cm and that no cancer cells were found in any nearby nodes.

References

[1] Rasheed M E H, Youseffi M, Jamil M M A and Rahman N A A 2021 *Medical Imaging and Analysis of Dense Breast Tissue: A Case Study* (Piscataway, NJ: IEEE)

[2] NHS UK 2020 *Consent and confidential patient information* (NHS UK) (https://nhsx.nhs.uk/information-governance/guidance/consent-and-confidential-patient-information/). Accessed 2020

[3] NHS UK 2019 *Genetic and genomic testing* (NHS UK) (https://nhs.uk/conditions/genetic-and-genomic-testing/). Accessed 2020

[4] NHS UK 2018 *Am I more at risk if my relatives have cancer?* (NHS UK) (https://nhs.uk/common-health-questions/lifestyle/am-i-more-at-risk-if-my-relatives-have-cancer/). Accessed 2020

[5] Chintamani C, Khandelwal R, Tandon M, Yashwant K, Kulshreshtha P, Aeron T, Bhatnagar D, Bansal A and Saxena S 2009 Carcinoma developing in a fibroadenoma in a woman with a family history of breast cancer: a case report and review of literature *Cases J.* **2** 9348

[6] Pilnik S 2003 *Common Breast Lesions: A Photographic Guide to Diagnosis and Treatment* (Cambridge: Cambridge University Press)

[7] Thigpen D, Kappler A and Brem R 2018 The role of ultrasound in screening dense breasts— a review of the literature and practical solutions for implementation *Diagnostics* **8** 20

[8] ACR ORG 2017 *ACR statement on reporting breast density in mammography reports and patient summaries* (ACR ORG) (https://acr.org/Advocacy-and-Economics/ACR-Position-Statements/Reporting-Breast-Density). Accessed 2020

[9] Shetty M 2015 *Breast Cancer Screening and Diagnosis: A Synopsis* (New York: Springer)

[10] breastcancer.org 2018 *Dense breasts* (breastcancer.org) (https://breastcancer.org/risk/factors/dense_breasts). Accessed 2018

[11] Cerrato F and Labow B 2013 Diagnosis and management of fibroadenomas in the adolescent breast *Semin. Plast. Surg.* **27** 23–5

[12] McMullen E, Zoumberos N and Kleer C 2019 Metaplastic breast carcinoma: update on histopathology and molecular alterations *Arch. Pathol. Lab. Med.* **143** 1492–6

[13] Jung S *et al* 2010 Worse prognosis of metaplastic breast cancer patients than other patients with triple-negative breast cancer *Breast Cancer Res. Treat.* **120** 627–37

[14] Wong W, Brogi E, Reis-Filho J, Plitas G, Robson M, Norton L, Morrow M and Wen H 2021 Poor response to neoadjuvant chemotherapy in metaplastic breast carcinoma *NPJ Breast Cancer* **7** 96

[15] Schwartz T, Mogal H, Papageorgiou C, Veerapong J and Hsueh E 2013 Metaplastic breast cancer: histologic characteristics, prognostic factors and systemic treatment strategies *Exp. Hematol. Oncol.* **2** 31

[16] 'What Is MpBC 2016 MpBC Global Alliance, Inc. (http://mpbcalliance.org/what-is-mpbc.html). Accessed 2021

[17] Mituś J, Sas-Korczyńska B, Kruczak A, Jasiówka M and Ryś J 2016 Metaplastic breast cancer with rapidly progressive recurrence in a young woman: case report and review of the literature *Arch. Med. Sci.* **12** 1384–8

[18] Reddy T, Rosato R, Li X, Moulder S, Piwnica-Worms H and Chang J 2020 A comprehensive overview of metaplastic breast cancer: clinical features and molecular aberrations *BCR* **22** 121

[19] He X, Ji J, Dong R, Liu H, Dai X, Wang C, Esteva F and Yeung S 2018 Prognosis in different subtypes of metaplastic breast cancer: a population-based analysis *Breast Cancer Res Treat.* **173** 329–41

[20] Feinstein A 1964 Monthly penicillin injections advised in rheumatic fever *JAMA* **190** 33

[21] Ralph A, Noonan S, Boardman C and Halkon C C B 2017 Prescribing for people with acute rheumatic fever *Aust Prescr.* **40** 70–5

[22] Gao Y, Shang Q, Li W, Guo W, Stojadinovic A, Mannion C, Man Y and Chen T 2020 Antibiotics for cancer treatment: a double-edged sword *J Cancer.* **11** 5135–49

[23] Petrelli F *et al* 2015 Use of antibiotics and risk of cancer: a systematic review and meta-analysis of observational studies *Cancers (Basel).* **11** 1174

[24] Velicer C, Heckbert S, Lampe J, Potter J, Robertson C and Taplin S 2004 Antibiotic use in relation to the risk of breast cancer *JAMA* **291** 827–35

[25] Bojinca V and Janta I 2012 Rheumatic diseases and malignancies *Maedica (Bucur).* **7** 364–71

[26] Cappelli L and Shah A 2020 The relationships between cancer and autoimmune rheumatic diseases *Best Pract. Res. Clin. Rheumatol.* **34** 101472

[27] Wyld L, Markopoulos C, Leidenius M and Senkus-Konefka E 2018 *Breast Cancer Management for Surgeons: A European Multidisciplinary Textbook* (Cham: Springer)

[28] NHS UK 2018 *Predictive genetic tests for cancer risk genes* (NHS UK) (https://nhs.uk/conditions/predictive-genetic-tests-cancer/). Accessed 2020

[29] Goutam M, Giriyapura C, Mishra S and Gupta S 2014 Titanium allergy: a literature review *Indian J Dermatol.* **59** 630

[30] Jain M, Lingarajah S, Luvsannyam E, Somagutta M, Jagani R, Sanni J, Ebose E, Tiesenga F and Jorge J 2021 Delayed titanium hypersensitivity and retained foreign body causing late abdominal complications *Case Rep. Surg.* **2021** 5515401

[31] Acton Q 2012 *Mitotic Inhibitors—Advances in Research and Application* 2012 edn (Atlanta: ScholarlyEditions)

[32] Koh J and Kim M 2019 Introduction of a new staging system of breast cancer for radiologists: an emphasis on the prognostic stage *Korean J. Radiol.* **20** 69–82

IOP Publishing

Breast Cancer and Medical Imaging

Mohammed Erkhawan Hameed Rasheed and Mansour Youseffi

Chapter 9

Discussion and conclusion

9.1 Discussion

The methodology selected for conducting the systematic review of the topics of breast cancer and medical imaging in this work presented an extensive review regarding all aspects of breast cancer and medical imaging. In regard to breast cancer, it included the breast anatomy (it is important to understand which parts of the breast are usually affected by breast cancer), the breast cancer stages, the risk factors of breast cancer such as family history and genetics, reproductive factors, as well as dietary and lifestyle behaviours. The current worldwide breast cancer prevention strategies used by healthcare providers are also presented in this work in addition to breast cancer symptoms, types of breast cancer, breast cancer incidence in men, in addition to the current breast cancer treatments provided around the globe for the treatment of patients with breast cancer including surgery, chemotherapy, radiotherapy and immunotherapy as part of biological therapy. Likewise, the systematic review also covered the topic of breast cancer recurrence and the available blood tests used for breast cancer recurrence prediction. Importantly, we include a systematic review of the topic of using complementary and alternative medicine for breast cancer and other types of cancer, which is believed to mainly work through boosting the body's natural immune system to kill the body's abnormal cells including the cancer cells. Similarly, this work also provided an extensive review regarding the medical imaging modalities used for the overall assessment of breast cancer such X-rays, mammograms, CT scans, USI, MRI, RI including PET and SPECT. The systematic review of past studies carried out in this work highlighted several examples of how hybrid modalities and their characteristics are integrated to improve and enhance combined medical images. The fusion of hybrid imaging techniques has been used as a way towards improving the specificity and sensitivity of these modalities to target medical images of breast cancer patients. The combination of different modalities has been subjected to address biological processes for better characterisation of the biology of tumours as well as for assessing cancer treatments and tumour responses and resistance. Among the significant fusion methods, a PET scan combined with a CT scan, PET scan combined with MRI, and SPECT scan combined with CT scan, all are known for their advantages and combined benefits. This work has revealed that the integration of imaging modalities for breast cancer has helped in assessing the importance of certain therapies in line with treatment planning and protocols. These improvements have further helped in sourcing the hard and soft tissues. Cancer diagnosis is the most critical step in the clinical process as oncologic assessments give significant importance to tumour detection and identifying the suspected as well as evident lesion areas. The cancer diagnosis process is divided into different sub-processes such as detection at an early stage, detection of malignancies at an advanced stage and detection at the progressive stage. However, the most effective diagnosing technique should be capable of responding to the range of risk factors, symptoms, stages of breast cancer and other variables associated with different cases. It can be depicted from the findings that breast cancer prevalence is associated with males and females, although the severity and intensity of the prevalence may vary. The evidence also highlighted the importance of age as an independent factor affecting the prevalence of breast cancer in women across the globe; however, an effective diagnostic technique should be capable of identifying the risk factors in women suffering from breast cancer, especially young women. This work has highlighted that, in addition to age, family history and genetics, hormone replacement therapy, birth control pills and alcohol consumption are significant risk factors associated with a higher prevalence of breast cancer. The analysis and critical review of recent studies has proved that mammography alone cannot be used as an effective modality in all populations of women, especially in women with dense breast tissue. Therefore, other modalities such as PET/CT, PET/MRI have been developed as improved methods for breast cancer imaging along with the traditional methods of X-rays, ultrasound, etc. When a PET scan technique is combined with other modalities such as MRI, it can produce remarkable results in the diagnosis phase of breast cancer assessment. Such assessment is necessary for the identification of effective treatments subsequently needed to deal with issues regarding patients with breast cancer. The outcome of this work has clearly concluded that the diagnostic stage must be capable of identifying all the underlying factors, i.e., not only the medical factors but also the sociodemographic and lifestyle factors. The diagnostic technique must also be capable of identifying the associated gene mutations responsible for the higher prevalence of breast cancer in women as highlighted in this work. The literature and the present study have identified some gene mutations as one of the high risk factors associated with breast cancer. Also, as explained in this work, diagnosis should be based and focused on deeper factors including differences in lifestyle such as obesity, alcohol consumption, diet, breast size and the associated risks. The image acquisition processing of some modalities such as PET makes it highly significant, specific and sensitive to the biologically active molecules and tissues found in the breast. Image acquisition protocol of the PET scan, which consists of the emission of gamma rays through a radionuclide tracer, is highly effective and functional and also it has operationally safe outcomes. Besides PET, ultrasound is also identified as effective in the diagnostic stage of breast cancer assessment. Automated improvements made in traditional ultrasound techniques have improved the efficiency of the image acquisition protocol and the image qualities. On the other hand, this investigation has also highlighted the overall sensitivity of MRI in producing breast cancer images. MRI has also been a popular method used for the diagnosis of breast cancer [1]. The importance of imaging surveillance after primary breast cancer treatment is also considered as an effective parameter in examining the different imaging techniques. Primary breast cancer treatment is related to the types of treatment strategies available for breast cancer patients such as surgery, chemotherapy, radiotherapy, hormone treatment and targeted therapies. This work has investigated the side effects of such therapies to consider/reflect on the recurrence of breast cancer after such treatments along with the management of side effects on a patient's overall health. Imaging surveillance after treatment is more complex and it must be capable of discriminating between the risk associated with complexities faced by patients afterwards. For this purpose, imaging techniques used at the treatment stage need to ensure whether the cancer has spread to other body parts, and if yes, whether or not it can be treated effectively through the consumption of cancer drugs. The results of the imaging technique must be capable of suggesting the treatment most likely to result in long lasting positive impact for patients. On the other hand, radionuclide imaging is identified as the most important technique for breast cancer imaging at the treatment stage. Among the modern medical imaging techniques, radionuclide imaging was identified as effective due to higher resolution features associated with breast cancer lesions. The characteristics of resolution and sensitivity further make it highly remarkable to produce effective results in the treatment stage. Clinical studies have confirmed that radionuclide imaging is an effective technique for the treatment stage as it is able to alter the treatment protocols developed in the initial assessment of breast cancer lesions [2]. The radionuclide imaging technique is not only capable of identifying the biological features but also is effective in detecting the functional features of the regions in the treatment stage. Researchers have also confirmed the significance of the radionuclide technique in identification of distant metastases staging for breast cancer patients, in the context of locally advanced, recurrent and metastasis disease. Furthermore, the radionuclide technique is highly effective in identifying the effects of breast cancer therapies. Both the first-time appearance and the relapse or recurrence of breast cancer are crucial for clinicians to deal with breast cancer patients. Breast cancer relapse can take place in two ways, local recurrence and cancer recurrence in other body parts. In the process of making effective identification of the type of recurrence, it is necessary for breast imaging techniques to differentiate initially among the different stages of cancer associated with such recurrence. While showing its compatibility in detecting different recurrences, radionuclide imaging has ultimately confirmed its effectiveness relative to other imaging techniques. Radionuclide imaging has also been used for tumour response modification for understanding the effects of treatments on disease resistance. In simple words, the technique has been in use for the protection of therapy responses as well as for controlling the progression of the disease in breast cancer patients [2].

Another medical imaging technique, mammography, has been identified in producing good quality medical images. Mammography can easily target lesions such as mass, mass with microcalcification, microcalcification, architectural distortion and local asymmetry. The effectiveness of the digital mammography technique has been improved and it is identified as a gold standard for breast cancer diagnosis. Mammography has the ability to provide adequate visualisation of soft tissue abnormalities. Soft tissues can lead to the development of benign tumours, which can occur at any part of the body. Effective imaging techniques, therefore, should be capable of identifying the appearance and behaviours of tumours in different body parts. Imaging techniques must be capable of understanding and differentiating aggressive and non-aggressive behaviours. Both the literature review as well as analysis of the different medical imaging techniques have confirmed that nuclear medicine advances are playing an important role in the detection of metastatic disease and support in the provision of complete information on soft tissue and bone metastases. It is also important to highlight that these techniques are capable of detecting information in a single scanning session without any need of repetitive scanning [2]. Follow-up surveillance should be more efficient compared to both the diagnosing and treatment stage imaging techniques. Follow-up imaging needs to revaluate all the factors responsible for the primary occurrence of breast cancer in order to ensure that they cannot lead to a relapse of the disease or slow down the process of treatment and interventions. Imaging modalities need to be responsive to the varying lengths and durations of the follow-up stage and should be capable of detecting early local recurrences or contralateral breast cancer, while evaluating and treating therapy-related complications such as menopausal symptoms, osteoporosis and the likelihood of second cancers and encourage breast cancer patients regarding the continuity of treatment [3]. The reviewed literature in this report has revealed that there are inadequate findings about the outcomes of medical imaging techniques, in particular due to lack of studies focusing on long-term outcomes. Such limited findings can be ultimately associated with the emergence of novel screening modalities, which have subsequently reduced the duration of the follow-up stages. The systematic review highlighting the recent studies has confirmed that clinical researchers are placing more effort in assessing the effectiveness of follow-up techniques related to breast cancer imaging. Breast cancer imaging has been initially assumed to be a diagnostic stage process. However, due to the emergence of the fusion-based modalities, examination of the effectiveness of existing medical imaging as well as new medical imaging techniques such as radionuclide imaging and medical image analysis modalities can be seen in recent studies. New nuclear imaging techniques have been increasingly investigated for the assessment of cancer patients including treatment response along with traditional medical imaging techniques. Investigations have revealed that MRI has proved itself as one of the most important imaging techniques, especially in dealing with young breast cancer patients and in cases of patients with dense breast tissue [4]. The use of the ultrasound imaging technique is also regarded as an effective modality, especially in dealing with invasive cancer types. Invasive cancers are highly complex and crucial due to varying levels of symptoms associated with their prevalence as well as their increased risk of spreading to other body parts and further worsening patients' situations. Follow-up imaging such as ultrasound can assist in identifying lobular invasive carcinomas. However, ultrasound is limited to local areas of the breast while detecting changes and recovery in the nipples, breast tissue, etc, while nuclear imaging techniques can detect tumours in other body parts too [2]. This work has highlighted ultrasound as an effective diagnostic technique for breast cancer imaging used across the globe. Besides ultrasound, MRI combined with the PET technique was also identified as the most widely used medical imaging modality due to its robust and comprehensive assessment of the cause as well as image acquisition approach. The systematic review revealed that the most effective diagnostic technique is the modality that is capable of detecting evident as well as suspicious breast lesions with a high level of sensitivity. The most effective diagnostic techniques are not affected by the small size of breast lesions, unexpected metabolic activity or changes in the microscopic tumour growth patterns. It is worth high-lighting that imaging techniques do not need only result-orienting abilities with respect to the specificity and sensitivity of medical images but they also should be responsive to the health and safety of patients too. Safety considerations are mostly related to the ability of imaging techniques to utilise contrast agents for addressing cancer-specific molecular markers. Imaging techniques are only effective when they are capable of reducing ionised radiation. The systematic review has highlighted that significant improvements have been made within the traditional ultrasound imaging technique, further making this imaging modality the most popular as well as the safest method to target different sizes of breast cancer lesions, irrespective of the size and density of the breast. Ultrasound is a safe and non-invasive method requiring few procedural preparations before conducting a diagnosis or follow-up examina-tion. Studies have also confirmed that the use of ultrasound in all stages of breast cancer assessment is very effective. It can be analysed that the most significant element in identifying the effectiveness of the technique is associated with the independence of the technique in targeting breast cancer in the diverse breast cancer population. The investigation has further confirmed the significance of soundwave frequency in targeting specific problematic lesion areas through the use of multiple colours and movements of frequencies. The technical, as well as procedural features of ultrasound, make it viable still among the novel medical imaging techniques. The arrival of more sensitive colour doppler and powerful machines have increased the efficiency of ultrasound in relation to the reduction of flowing solid masses and for the differ-entiation of flow. Ultrasound, in comparison to the other techniques, is effective in identifying the management issues as well as normal tissues associated with breast lesions. It is also capable of detecting the surrounding stiffness [5]. Positron emission tomography combined with magnetic resonance imaging is a hybrid imaging technology that has also confirmed the potential of finding soft tissue and functional imaging aspects related to breast cancer assessment. Besides breast examination, PET/ MRI was also identified as effective for whole-body assessment. The functionality provided by the tracers of the PET technique is the further examination of molecular, functional, as well as anatomical information. Simultaneous acquisition of breast data using PET/MRI functionalities and preparations have also confirmed that it is an innovative technology which is able to produce exceptional quality images that are conclusive evidence with low variations. All assessment outcomes can be easily achieved in one single exam without the need of immediate measures [6]. The use of the qualitative as well as quantitative information about the medical imaging techniques has reported the significance and importance of this investigation. The literature review includes recent studies describing the role of different modalities in the diagnosis, treatment and follow-up stages of breast cancer. A large set of imaging modalities was reviewed in the current investigation including both traditional methods as well as novel techniques. There is a possibility that a wide range of studies is now available for traditional methods such as ultrasound, MRI, mammography while in comparison very few studies have been initially conducted by researchers for the modern and normal imaging techniques such as CT, MRI and radionuclide imaging. Likewise, it can be discussed that for different modalities a number of studies were used to assess their role at different stages of breast cancer assessment. The variation in the sample sizes was due to the availability of the studies related to the imaging techniques. For the traditional techniques, the bulk of academic studies were available for the diagnosis stage while a small number of studies were found for the other stages. For this reason, sample size can be related to the differences in the weightage given to the discussion of the different medical imaging techniques. It is observed that some of the techniques were precisely discussed due to the small number of studies found for the assessment. In a similar context, the examination and assessment of follow-up imaging techniques were quite low due to more focus by researchers being on the diagnostic and treatment stages. The current investigation has highlighted the most effective medical imaging technique for breast cancer imaging, and the findings are also helpful in suggesting the need to improve the functional as well as safety-related features for improving the effectiveness of breast cancer imaging modalities. Preference has been given to those imaging techniques which require less effort and at the same time produce better outcomes. Clinical experts have also changed their demands in relation to the effectiveness of medical imaging capable of producing high-quality images by protecting the health of their patients. It is realised that some of the medical imaging techniques are still able to produce harmful effects on the physical aspects of breast cancer lesions. Therefore, regardless of the improvements in medical imaging modalities that have been accomplished, as in the case of the hybrid approach, the effectiveness of the technique is still reliant on the ability to produce safe images.

9.2 Conclusion

In conclusion, and based on the present evidence-based discussions that compare past studies in recent years, more improvements have been evidenced in the medical imaging field such as enhancement of the image acquisition protocols as well as increased safety of patients. In summary, from the key insights gathered from this investigation of the role of medical imaging techniques in the overall assessment of breast cancer, the main points are related to the effective medical imaging modality that can be used effectively in the diagnosis, treatment, as well as in the follow-up stages for assessment of breast cancer as highlighted in this work. In this work, a review of the traditional and modern medical imaging techniques has confirmed the improvements undertaken by healthcare professionals and clinicians in enhancing the ability of imaging techniques to diagnose, treat and monitor the recurrences of breast cancer in the overall population of breast cancer patients. However, such effectiveness of these imaging techniques cannot be assessed without relating it to the risk factors, symptoms and patients' demographic attributes such as age, prevention strategies, treatment options and the physical attributes of the breast. Sociodemographic variables of patients such as age, lifestyle, and genetics and hereditary conditions have to be considered while using any medical imaging technique. Multi-level factors are required to be considered while assessing the effectiveness of any modular approach. Deeper analysis of the physical changes appearing in the breasts and breast parts as well as the risk factors behind it, specifically the gene mutation involved, are also essential to be considered while assessing effectiveness. A detailed overview of breast cancer, its various stages and different factors associated with such stages need to be considered for gaining a classification of the imaging techniques suitable for different stages of breast cancer imaging. The systematic review conducted in this work has confirmed the use of new technologies such as the fusion of different modalities in increasing the overall assessment and monitoring of the disease. A range of medical imaging modalities, for example, X-ray, mammography, CT, ultrasound, MRI, PET and radionuclide imaging, were reviewed in this work for assessing the effectiveness required to acquire an image. Besides reviewing the image acquisition protocols for these medical imaging techniques, consideration was also made of their safety and health issues. This work has confirmed ultrasound as the most effective technique that can be used in all three stages of breast cancer assessment. Image acquisition protocol of ultrasound imaging has helped in enhancing the ability to deal with breast cancer cases and in decreasing the mortality rate caused by breast cancer. This work has confirmed the focus on increasing the features of medical imaging techniques in order to make it crucial for the treatment planning and strategic purpose such as the use of many fusion-based techniques, for example, PET with CT and PET with MRI. Treatment of breast cancer requires a critical approach towards the technical as well as the functional and biological features to target the affected breast cells and the use of techniques which can help in altering the path of the treatment protocols according to the effects of individual cases. Such alterations and modifications are further required to be aligned with the severity of the risk factors and the side effects of treatments. The imaging techniques contributing vitally to relating the patient-related factors with other medical factors in order to detect the appropriate imaging technique. These imaging techniques at different stages of breast cancer screening, when applied adequately, are capable of leading to an effective physical as well as psychological recovery. This work has critically discussed that researchers have mainly focused on the diagnosis and treatment stages, whereas the follow-up stage is not given much significance and sufficient attention. This work has also shown that follow-up cannot be separated from the physical perspective. Long-term survivorship of breast cancer patients needs to be addressed through responsiveness to the challenges faced by the researchers in the context of patients' expectations after the completion of treatment.

Follow-up screening is therefore as crucial as the diagnosis and treatment stages in order to investigate the side effects of the treatment as well as long-term implications of living with breast cancer. Therefore, an effective screening technique needs to concentrate on the follow-up care procedure along with the diagnosis and treatment. This work has highlighted that a single screening method or dual screening technique must be used for routine stage evaluation at the early breast cancer phase and evaluation of the functional and anatomical information in the advanced stages. This work has informed the reader that different screening techniques are capable of dealing with the issues at pre- as well as post-operative procedures and therefore the screening procedure needs to be considered in the staging and management of local recurrence and loco-regional disease appearances. This work has also confirmed that the high-level effectiveness and the characteristics of all the imaging techniques are needed to be combined or integrated for new formation in all stages of the assessment rather than only focusing on one specific imaging stage. The improved technique needs to be useful in the identification of the clear as well as suspected affected areas despite the effects of size, metabolic activity, subtype, growth of the tumour and proliferation. The effective technique is also capable of providing information targeted by medical experts along with the provision of additional information about the unsuspected distant metathesis. The sensitivity as well as specificity of the modality should be clearly directed towards detection as well as assessment of breast lesions in dense breasts as well as in the follow-up stages of the disease. The findings of the work have also highlighted a specific point related to the use of image acquisition protocols, i.e., the scanner, tracer or any other instrument to be used for capturing images of the cancerous tissues (active) or other body areas (non-active) should be user-friendly and security-oriented for patients. It is therefore necessary to assess the effectiveness of medical imaging techniques by looking into the benefits and risks of each technique. It is hoped that these findings will provide significant benefits in understanding the possible occurrence of cancer due to environmental gene mutations and preventive strategies, thus making a huge difference to wellbeing and the avoidance of unhealthy conditions and as a whole to the related scientific communities including the medical imaging modalities. Irrespective of the availability of numerous studies of medical imaging techniques used for breast cancer screening, diagnosis and treatment monitoring, the way is still open for further development in order to identify one specific modality fulfilling all purposes. This investigation has highlighted traditional as well as modern imaging techniques used by biomedical engineers and clinicians as well as other healthcare professionals for the effective assessment of breast cancer patients at different stages of the disease, i.e., the early stages as well as the advanced stages. Through detailed descriptive and systematic assessment of different imaging techniques covered in this work, including image composition protocols, and their ability to contribute towards human health and safety, this work has presented some improvements that have been made to medical imaging techniques used for diagnosing patients with breast cancer, including work that has been done on targeting dense breasts by improving image quality as well as the size of various images. The role of effective imaging can therefore be attributed towards the decline in breast cancer mortality rates across the globe.

9.3 Recommendations

From the conclusions drawn in this work, ultrasound and PET with MRI were identified as the most effective techniques that can help clinicians in the overall assessment of breast cancer and in respect to screening, diagnosis and treatment monitoring of the disease. These findings can be implemented to conduct future experimental studies based on randomised controlled trials. These trials can substantiate the effectiveness of ultrasound and PET with the MRI fusion technique by conducting practical experiments with breast cancer patients. It is therefore suggested that future trials are conducted by considering the effectiveness of the imaging techniques in the overall assessment, i.e., stage-based assessment. It is also recommended that researchers carry out such investigations by using two different groups such as a breast cancer patient group and control group. Comparative assessment of the patient group with the control group would effectively identify the strengths, weaknesses as well as the limitations in using these techniques for breast cancer assessment.

9.4 Implications

The findings of the current work have significant implications on the theoretical as well as practical aspects related to this work. The in-depth analysis of past studies and the systematic review have provided grounds for the assessment of different medical imaging modalities available to be used for breast cancer assessment in detail. The findings of this work have also allowed the differentiation of different traditional as well as modern techniques to highlight the improvements evolving in the imaging field. The systematic review is an important addition to the available scientific literature. The points mentioned regarding image acquisition protocols, technical aspects, as well as safety-related aspects will be helpful for researchers to realise the areas needed for improvement regarding different medical imaging techniques.

References

[1] cancerresearchuk.org 2020 *Breast MRI scan* (cancerresearchuk.org) (https://cancerresearchuk.org/about-cancer/breast-cancer/getting-diagnosed/tests-diagnose/breast-mri-scan). Accessed May 2020
[2] Surti S 2014 Radionuclide methods and instrumentation for breast cancer detection and diagnosis *Semin. Nucl. Med.* **4** 271–80
[3] cancer.org 2019 *Follow up care after breast cancer treatment* (cancer.org). (https://cancer.org/cancer/breast-cancer/living-as-a-breast-cancer-survivor/follow-up-care-after-breast-cancer-treatment.html). Accessed May 2020
[4] Bakker M, de Lange S V, Pijnappel R and Mann R 2019 Supplemental MRI screening for women with extremely dense breast tissue *New Engl. J. Med.* **381** 2091–102
[5] Ibrahim R, Rahmat K, Fadzli F, Rozalli F, Westerhout C, Alli K, Vijayananthan A and Moosa F 2016 Evaluation of solid breast lesions with power Doppler: value of penetrating vessels as a predictor of malignancy *Singap. Med. J.* **57** 634–40
[6] Umutlu L and Herrmann K 2018 *PET/MR Imaging: Current and Emerging Applications* (New York: Springer)

www.ingramcontent.com/pod-product-compliance
Lightning Source LLC
Chambersburg PA
CBHW082107210326
41599CB00033B/6622